The
Clinical
Nurse
Specialist

Perspectives on Practice

The Clinical Nurse Specialist

Perspectives on Practice

Edited by

Shirley W. Menard M.S.N., R.N., C.P.N.P.

Assistant Professor of Clinical Nursing
Clinical Nurse Specialist
University of Texas Health Science Center School of Nursing
Medical Center Hospital
San Antonio, Texas

A WILEY MEDICAL PUBLICATION
JOHN WILEY & SONS

New York • Chichester • Brisbane • Toronto • Singapore

Library of Congress Cataloging in Publication Data:

The clinical nurse specialist.

(A Wiley medical publication)
Includes bibliographies and index.
1. Nurse practitioners.   I. Menard, Shirley W.
II. Series. [DNLM: 1. Nurse Clinicians.   WY 128 C6405]
RT82.8.C575 1987   610.73'0692   86-19117
ISBN 0-471-87050-1

Printed in the United States of America

10 9 8 7 6 5 4 3 2

*This book is dedicated
to my hope for the future —*

my daughter, Christina Rose Menard

CONTRIBUTORS

ELEANOR ADASKIN, M.A., R.N., Clinical Nurse Specialist/Psychiatry, St. Boniface General Hospital, Winnepeg, Canada, Doctoral Candidate in Nursing, University of Texas, Austin, Texas

BARBARA CARLILE-HOLMES, M.S.N., R.N., Oncology Clinical Nurse Specialist, University of Texas Health Science Center Medical School, San Antonio, Texas

SUSAN COONING, M.S., R.N., Assistant Professor of Clinical Nursing, Clinical Nurse Specialist, University of Texas Health Science Center at San Antonio School of Nursing, Santa Rosa Children's Hospital, San Antonio, Texas

NANCY GIRARD, M.S.N., C.R.N., R.N., Assistant Professor of Clinical Nursing, Clinical Nurse Specialist, University of Texas Health Science Center at San Antonio School of Nursing, Medical Center Hospital, San Antonio, Texas

EVELYN L. GONZALES, M.S.N., R.N., Assistant Clinical Professor, UCLA School of Nursing, Los Angeles, California

DIANA HUSTON-ANDERSON, M.S.N., R.N., Clinical Nurse Specialist/Arthritis, St. Paul Medical Center, Dallas, Texas

ANNIE JOHNY, M.S., R.N., Director of Clinical Nurse Specialists, St. Paul Medical Center, Dallas, Texas

JULIE S. MEYER, M.S.N., R.N., Assistant Professor of Clinical Nursing, Clinical Nurse Specialist, University of Texas Health Science Center at San Antonio School of Nursing, Medical Center Hospital, San Antonio, Texas

CHRISTY A. PRICE, M.S.N., R.N., Clinical Nurse Specialist/Renal, San Diego Naval Hospital, San Diego, California

JOAN M. WABSCHALL, M.S., R.N., Head Nurse, Children's Hospital Emergency Services, Santa Rosa Medical Center, San Antonio, Texas

FOREWORD

Patients need help. Patients need information. Patients need the best nursing care available. As these needs in hospitals and homes become more complex and as the care patients receive increases in sophistication, the education and knowledge of the person they turn to for help and information also needs to be specialized and timely. Nursing has recognized that an individual with advanced education, experience, and commitment is needed in all areas of today's health care system to work with patients, families, nursing and medical staff, and students in the health professions. The title given to this person has been clinical nurse specialist (CNS), denoting the special skills of the nurse in a clinical area of expertness. The CNS is finding a wide gap in nursing that needs filling. Filling this gap necessitates assuming multiple roles and responsibilities and also developing and marketing these roles in unique and creative ways.

The history of the CNS is short, and yet the need is great within the health care delivery system. Creating a demand is going to be a key to the future growth of this specialist. The demand also needs to be coupled with cost-effectiveness studies. Effecting quality care is a goal and an achievement but not a salable goal in the for-profit health care system.

The American Nurses Association has supported the development of the CNS category by developing standards of practice that incorporate the CNSs' nurse activities. Practicing CNSs are also strong enough in numbers to work together to educate the industry in relation to the effectiveness of hiring CNSs. Books such as this one will help encourage nurses to move into CNS roles and help other nurses understand the role so it can be interpreted to colleagues in the health professions.

Combining clinical activities, education, consultation, and research into one job is difficult, and yet many nurses are attempting to follow this model and are extremely effective in all phases of their activity. They are demonstrating that it can be done, is being done, and is a highly successful role within nursing practice. The contributors to this book have outlined specific roles, activities, and strategies to assist in being an effective CNS. It is an excellent guidebook for nurses contemplating this role.

Nursing and nurses are having a significant impact on the care and recovery of patients. Nurses with expert knowledge in areas of specialization are crucial to the future advancement of quality patient care. Patients need help and information and the skilled care of the CNS. May the tribe increase!

PATTY L. HAWKEN, PH.D., R.N.
Dean, School of Nursing

University of Texas
Health Science Center
San Antonio, Texas

PREFACE

The knowledge and expertise that a clinical nurse specialist (CNS) brings to the health care team can be vital to the quality of patient care. Nursing service administrators who include CNSs on the nursing care team very quickly identify the contributions these expert clinicians make not only to patient care but also to staff education and morale.

Graduate nursing students have long needed a text that can help them transform theory into the real world of the CNS. The beginning CNS frequently has no role model or peers to whom she can turn for guidance in her practice.* The experienced CNS may wish to refresh her knowledge concerning a specific role or function. Hospital administrators and nursing administrators have a need to understand the many-faceted roles of the CNS so as to better appreciate what the CNS may offer to the institution.

The purpose of this book is to bridge the gap between theory and practice for the CNS, and through discussion of the roles of the CNS and other current issues, to clarify ways in which the CNS can effectively and efficiently contribute to the health care team. The book examines the theory behind the issues and then demonstrates practical, realistic steps for the CNS to implement a specific role successfully.

The text begins by examining the framework by which to consider the practice of the CNS. Historical perspectives, development of the role, marketing of the CNS, and power, politics, and leadership all play a significant part of this backdrop. The primary roles of the CNS—that of practitioner, teacher, consultant, and researcher are then examined. In these as in other chapters, practical aspects of implementation are reinforced by actual case studies. In addition, one chapter is devoted to appropriate evaluation of the CNS's worth and performance level. The final chapter examines a few of the possibilities awaiting the CNS, and is meant to spark the interest of the CNS to develop creative methods of practice.

*In the interest of time and ease for the reader, the term *she* will be used to refer to the CNS, and *he* will be used to refer to the patient/client.

The future of the CNS is open to many exciting possibilities. It is my hope that *The Clinical Nurse Specialist: Perspectives on Practice* will contribute to those possibilities by serving as a handbook for beginning CNSs, as a text for graduate students in nursing, as a resource for experienced CNSs and other master's-prepared practitioners, and as a guide for administrators to encourage implementation and support of the CNS role.

SHIRLEY W. MENARD

San Antonio, Texas
December 1986

ACKNOWLEDGMENTS

This section very appropriately comes at the beginning because there could be no book without the help and encouragement of family, colleagues, and friends.

My love and appreciation go first to my husband, Frenchie, and our daughter, Christina. As deadlines approached, they lived with someone who had little time to talk, listen, or cook. They helped me remain sane.

This book really began at the encouragement of two nurses I call mentors, colleagues, and friends. I am truly lucky to have been exposed to the fine role modeling of Glenda Butnarescu, M.S.N., R.N., and Marie McGrath, Ph.D., R.N. They supported me through some difficult times.

I am extremely grateful for the support of my two "bosses," Patty Hawken, Ph.D., R.N., Dean, School of Nursing, The University of Texas Health Science Center at San Antonio, and Nora Wilson, M.S., R.N., Associate Administrator for Patient Care, Medical Center Hospital, San Antonio, Texas.

To all of my colleagues and friends at The University of Texas Health Science Center and Medical Center Hospital, thanks for all of the help and interest.

Typing a manuscript is never easy, but Ann Morrison and Peg Campbell did it quickly and efficiently. Peg also did a fine job of editing the draft.

This book went through a number of crises as any developing book will. I cannot thank Jane de Groot, editor at John Wiley & Sons, enough for her fine guidance. Most of all, I found a good friend.

S.W.M.

CONTENTS

The
Clinical
Nurse
Specialist

Perspectives on Practice

1

THE CNS: HISTORICAL PERSPECTIVES

Shirley W. Menard, M.S.N., R.N.

Chapter Objectives

At the conclusion of this chapter, the reader will:

1. Understand the relationship cf nursing history to the development of the clinical nurse specialist (CNS) role.
2. Be familiar with the contributions of selected nurses to the expanded nursing role.

The future of nursing has always been seen in its past; therefore, no book on clinical specialization would be complete without a look at the history of the subject. Although the actual history of clinical specialization began in the 1940s with Peplau and later with Reiter (Peplau, 1965), there were many events that occurred prior to that time that have influenced the expanding role of nursing. This chapter will look at social and economic historical events as well as at nursing history in an attempt to show how our past has influenced our present.

Although Florence Nightingale was not a clinical specialist, she certainly introduced some concepts basic to the role. She was respected for her clinical and administrative skills as well as her ability to teach others. She was assertive and knew how to find and use power. During the Crimean War, nurses had to ally themselves with physicians in order to obtain their objective, which was caring for wounded soldiers (Nightingale, 1860).

In the United States, a widespread use of nurses, whether in an expanded role or not, was not possible due to many social and economic factors. Additionally, there were simply not enough *trained* nurses. Women who had graduated from a school of nursing were highly sought after by patients for private duty. In fact, they became our first really autonomous practitioners. In this sense, many of the early nurses were practicing in what could be considered an expanded role.

The late 1800s saw several events that had an impact on nursing. In 1864, a Nursing Bureau was established in Washington with its major emphasis the establishment of training schools for nurses in principal cities. At about the same time (1869), the National Women's Suffrage Association was organized to promote voting rights for women. Lavinia Dock, a nurse, was an early supporter of this movement. She saw women's rights as a way to promote and expand the rights of nurses. (Kelly, 1976, p. 46). Although Ms. Dock tried very hard to involve nurses in the women's suffrage movement, full support was not ever completely obtained.

When discussing early expanded roles, the name of Lillian Wald usually arises. Ms. Wald founded the Henry Street Settlement in New York City. Nurses working out of the Settlement House were autonomous to a great extent. They also performed many of the roles one sees in the modern clinical nurse specialist (CNS). They were skilled practitioners and confident patient educators. Certainly they were change agents in that their practice changed not only the lives of their patients but also nursing itself.

Because higher education is a part of clinical specialization, it is appropriate to look at early education for nurses. The first training school for nurses was established at New England Hospital for Women and Children with Linda Richards as its first graduate in 1872 (Anderson, 1981, p. 22). The University of Texas established a school of nursing as a regular division of its medical department in 1894. However, the University of Minnesota had the first autonomous university nursing program. In 1899, Teachers College in New York was the first to offer courses (in hospital economics) to graduate nurses. Columbia granted the first graduate nursing degree in 1909. Advanced clinical nurses in the 1950s went to the universities for higher education, and by the 1960s, all post basic education for specialization in clinical nursing was provided in graduate programs. The first such CNS program was established at Rutgers in 1954 by Peplau (Smoyak, 1976, p. 679).

Between 1900 and 1930, nursing was becoming established in the United States. Medical knowledge was also expanding, and nurses began moving into new positions. In 1902, Linda Rogers became the first nurse to work in a public school system. Clara Weeks wrote the first nursing text in 1900. The first joint practice was at Massachusetts General Hospital in 1905 when Medical Social Service was begun by Dr. Richard C. Cabot with Ida M. Cannon, a nurse, his associate (Kelly, 1975, p. 70).

The Spanish American War and World War I increased the need for highly skilled nurses, and military nursing was begun. The year 1920 brought the ratification of the Nineteenth Amendment, giving women the right to vote.

Mary Breckenridge began the Frontier Nursing Service in Kentucky in the 1920s and with it gave nurses a chance to step into a truly expanded role. These nurses were responsible in large part for the reduction in maternal and infant mortality in that area of the country. The Frontier Nursing Service stands today as a leader in expanded roles for nurses.

The first reference to the role of the clinical specialist was made by Peplau in the 1940s when psychiatric clinical nurse specialists first came on the scene. Frances Reiter used the term *nurse clinician* in 1943 and also traced the role back to the early 1900s (Reiter, 1966, p. 274). World War II saw military nursing expand its scope and also saw the downswing of private-duty nursing. During World War II, nurses were utilized heavily by the military so there were fewer nurses available for civilian needs. Following World War II, more hospitals were built, and health insurance became available; the number of nurses working in hospitals rose and thus began giving up their autonomy to become employees. Advances in medical technology and more sophisticated therapeutic regimens required that patients be hospitalized, and nurses were needed to monitor patients' progress. Other members joined the health care team, including licensed vocational nurses, social workers, dieticians, physical therapists, occupational therapists, and others. Care was beginning to fragment, and someone was needed to coordinate care. The role of the CNS seemed to result from the frustration that nurses felt over the fragmentation of patient care (Bullough & Bullough, 1977, p. 5).

In 1950, a code of ethics was adopted by the American Nurses Association. This led to standards of nursing care from which not only CNSs but all nurses could practice. The American Nurses Association model statement on the definition of nursing was introduced in 1955 (Bullough & Bullough, 1978) and was utilized by many states in revisions of state nurse practice acts.

Clinical specialization as a concept was formalized in 1956 at the National

Working Conference on the Education of the Clinical Specialist in Psychiatric Nursing, which was held in Williamsburg, Virginia. Participants at the conference "set a primary goal of improving nursing care through rehabilitation, prevention and promotion of positive health in addition to cure" (Kuntz et al., 1980, p. 90). This was the first meeting with an emphasis on clinical specialization.

The Korean conflict brought many changes in the type of patients seen in hospitals. Helicopters were used to transport wounded soldiers from the front to Mobile Army Surgical Hospital (MASH) units, where they could be treated and stabilized before being sent to Japan or the United States for long-term care. Triage and the immediate use of available technology and techniques contributed to the salvaging of patients who previously would have died. This kind of treatment meant that hospital personnel cared for extremely critical patients. Due to procedural and technological advances, civilian hospitals were also seeing more critically ill patients. External cardiac massage had been developed prior to 1950 but only began to be widely taught and used in the late 1950s and early 1960s. Cardiac patients who would have died were now being saved, and special equipment and skills were needed to care for these patients. Nursing care became more involved as more complex patients were seen.

There were many events in the 1960s that helped to shape the future of nursing and especially clinical specialization. The Vietnam War began early in the 1960s and took nurses to Southeast Asia. Due to increased technology, casualties were evacuated from the battlefields to the MASH units in a matter of minutes. Nurses were responsible for very high level care of severely injured patients. These same nurses came back to civilian hospitals with advanced skills and abilities. Many of these nurses found that they were not able to practice to the full extent of their abilities due to a more restricted view of nursing in civilian hospitals.

In 1962, a coronary care unit was opened at Bethany Hospital in Kansas City, Kansas (Bullough & Bullough, 1978, p. 204). As nurses and physicians had to work closely together in these units, they began to collaborate on the care their patients received. Also in 1962, at Massachusetts General Hospital, nurses were totally responsible for the care of chronically ill patients in the outpatient department. Expanded roles were beginning to come into their own.

One of the major reasons that nurses were unable to advance either professionally or economically dealt with general attitudes toward women and minorities. The Civil Rights Act in 1964 led the way for civil rights of many groups to be realized. The late 1960s also saw the beginning of the women's movement, which culminated in the formation of the National Organization of Women (NOW). In the early suffrage movement (as stated previously), Lavinia Dock urged nurses to join their sisters, but nurses did not heed Ms. Dock. Early in the women's movement, nurses began to see that the only way to change their situation was by joining forces similar to NOW. The time was ripe to change paternalistic attitudes present too long in hospitals.

In a position paper in 1965, the ANA declared that the title CNS should be used only by nurses with a master's degree in nursing (M.S.N., M.N., M.S.) or higher (ANA, 1965). The professional association was once again trying to establish an educational basis for entry into a specific practice. Although the battle for entry level into basic professional nursing practice is still an issue, many nurses now believe that a graduate degree is needed to enter specialty practice.

The 1970s saw a dramatic rise in medical technology and in the number of both general and specialized intensive care units. A nationwide physician shortage created increased demands on nurses both inside and outside the hospital. Nurses took on many technical procedures that physicians had been doing, such as chemotherapy and sophisticated monitoring systems. This increased role for nurses raised legal questions that only substantial changes in state practice acts could answer. The discussion goes on in state legislatures today.

The Equal Rights Amendment was begun in 1971 in an effort to disallow discrimination on the basis of sex. Women began to have changing roles with increased assertiveness and a quest for egalitarianism. In April 1973, Nurses NOW was formed in Pittsburgh, Pennsylvania, to help put forth the nurse's role in the women's movement.

In 1971, the Secretary of Health, Education and Welfare formed an interdisciplinary committee to study potential and actual new roles for nursing. The report from this committee (U.S. Department of HEW, 1971, p. 2) stated:

> We believe that the future of nursing must encompass a substantially larger place within the community of the health professionals. Moreover, we believe that extending the scope of nursing practice is essential if this nation is to achieve the goal of equal access to health services for all its citizens. . . .

This report went on to suggest that professional education should demonstrate the physician–nurse team concept; that there should be national commonalities in state practice acts; that these should be collaborative programs within schools; and that to measure impact in health care delivery, a cost analysis should be done. Another report, the Lysaught Report, dealt with nursing education and came out of the National Commission for the Study of Nursing and Nursing Education (Lysaught, 1970). It stated that master planning for graduate nursing education must be concerned with the number and type of graduate programs. It suggested that priority should go to programs preparing faculty, *master clinicians*, and nurse administrators.

The 1970s and early 1980s saw the rise of clinical specialization. Specialized units have proliferated necessitating more educated and experienced nurses. More hospitals began hiring CNSs, but frequently there was little peer support within the hospital. Nationally, three things have happened to give the CNS the peer support she needs. National certifying examinations for generalized and specialized areas of practice were begun by ANA (as well as other organizations) around 1975. In 1980, the Congress for Nursing Practice, American Nurses Association, published a lengthy statement on nursing practice. It included a description of CNS education, roles, functions, and needs (ANA, 1980, pp. 21–29). This description helps the CNS to know who her peers are so that she can seek out those people. The third event was the formation of the Council of Clinical Nurse Specialists in 1982. Under the leadership of Ann Hamric from Illinois, this council has rapidly grown and has participated in sponsoring major conferences for CNSs. Councils are also being formed under local and/or state nursing associations. As CNSs gather together, they are able to gain strength from each other and solve common problems.

What does the future hold for clinical nurse specialization? It would appear that as the CNS continues to contribute to high quality and cost-effective patient care, hospitals will continue to utilize the CNS. In these difficult economic times, the pressure is on CNSs to concretely show their cost-effectiveness and maintain high levels of education and experience.

BIBLIOGRAPHY

American Nurses Association. (1980). Nursing: A social policy statement. New York: American Nurses Association.

American Nurses Association. (1971, November). Extending the scope of nursing practice: A report of the secretary's committee to study extended roles for nurses. Washington, DC:U.S. Department, HEW.

American Nurses Association. (1965). Educational preparation for nurse practitioners and assistants to nurses: A position paper. New York: American Nurses Association.

Aiken, L. (Ed.). (1982). *Nursing in the 80's: Crises, opportunities, challenges.* Philadelphia: Lippincott.

Amenta, M. (1977). NURSES NOW: A model of worksite organizing. *Nursing Forum,*
16(3,4), 343–345.

Anderson, N. (1981, January). The historical development of American nursing education. *Journal of Nursing Education,* **20**(1), 18–31.

Bullough, B., & Bullough, V. (1977). *Expanding horizons for nurses.* New York:
Springer.

Bullough, B., & Bullough, V. (1978). *The care of the sick: The emergence of modern
nursing.* New York: Springer.

Flanagan, L. (1979). *One strong voice, the story of the American Nurses Association,*
Vol. 1 (pp. 10–663). St. Louis: American Journal of Nursing Publishers.

Gowers, S. (1981, May 20). Something special. *Nursing Mirror,* **152**(2), 30–31.

Kalisch, P., & Kalisch, B. (1980). *The history of American nursing.* Boston: Little,
Brown.

Kelly, L.Y. (1975). *Dimensions of professional nursing* (3rd ed.) (pp. 62–84, 93–95, &
473–747). New York: MacMillan.

Kelly, L.Y. (1976, October). Our nursing heritage: Have we renounced it? *Image,*
8(3), 43–48.

Kuntz, S., Stehle, J., & Marshall, R. (1980). The psychiatric clinical specialist: The
progression of a specialty. *Perspectives in Psychiatric Care,* **17**(2), 90–92.

Lamb, S. (1981). The role of nurse clinicians in current practice. *Journal of Neuro-
surgical Nursing,* **11**(3), 156–159.

Lysaught, J. (1970). *National commission for the study of nursing and nursing education.* New York: McGraw-Hill.

Nightingale, F. (1860). *Notes on nursing: What it is and what it is not.* London: Harrison and Sons.

Peplau, H. (1965, August). Specialization in professional nursing. *Nursing Science,*
3, 268–287.

Reiter, F. (1966). The nurse-clinician. *American Journal of Nursing,* **66**, 274–280.

Smith, F. (1981, May). Florence Nightingale: Early feminist. *American Journal of
Nursing,* **81**(5), 1021–1024.

Smoyak, S.A. (1976, November). Specialization in nursing: From then to now. *Nursing Outlook,* **24**(11), 676–681.

White, N. (1978, May). ERA: The chance for equality. *Nursing Administration Quarterly,* **3** 79–81.

2

THE CNS: DEVELOPMENT OF THE ROLE

Nancy Girard, M.S.N., R.N., C.S.

Chapter Objectives

At the conclusion of this chapter the reader will:

1. Recognize the definition of *role* and its development.
2. Relate role development to nursing and to the clinical nurse specialist (CNS).
3. Define the major roles, along with problems of those roles.
4. Discuss the way in which change agent is incorporated into other CNS roles.

Funk and Wagnall's standard dictionary defines *role* as: "A part or character taken by an actor: any assumed character or function" (1960). The word is a noun, which is a first-order description of someone or something that performs an action.

The nursing literature does not agree to a single definition of the word *role*. Instead, there is a composite of meanings that have been derived through the years. Nursing articles use the word as a noun, verb, or characteristics, such as role model, role function, or role conflict. This terminology difference may increase the confusion in trying to define and explain the CNS's functions in today's society. Used as defined, *role* (n) accurately describes the CNS as a person of action who accomplishes something. This chapter will review role development and will discuss various aspects of the roles of the CNS today.

NURSING ROLE DEVELOPMENT

Much of the information about role development that nursing identifies with today comes from other sciences. In 1936, role was described by social psychologists as the actions or functions that must be done by a person to prove the position that they held in society or in their occupations (Linton, 1936). Roles were seen as functions that defined the person's status, occupation, and behavior in a specific society. Some authors stated that roles contain and restrain behavior and help set guidelines for normal social and work behavior (Miller, 1963; Biddle & Thomas, 1966). Roles were tied closely to certain identifiable positions in society, such as age, sex, family, status, occupation, and social groupings (Linton, 1945). Role functions could be attained by personal effort, or were uncontrolled, such as age or sex of the individual.

Individual articles in nursing literature have attempted to describe role for many years. In 1959, the *American Journal of Nursing* published articles about nursing's role conflict and confusion. Professional nursing organizations such as the National League of Nursing (NLN) discussed the nurse's role as employee. Even the government tried to define the role of the nurse in a 1972 publication on expanded roles (HEW). Today, nursing's role is still evolving. Nurses are better educated and more independent in their assessment and knowledge of patient care needs. Also, more men are entering the career field.

However, parallel to nursing's perception of a change occurring in their role functions is the frequent opinion of others in the health care field that it remain unchanged. Hospitals and other health care institutions hire nurses as employees, so their defined functions still identify their status. Therefore, confusion for today's nurse often occurs when the employer retains society's older definition of the functions of a nurse and the nurse has visions of new and expanded roles.

CNS ROLE DEVELOPMENT

The roles, or functions and characteristics, of the CNS developed along theoretical lines described in social and psychological fields. In 1965, Hildegard Peplau talked of societal trends that were then leading nurses into specialization, with the primary role being that of expert caregiver. She also mentioned other roles such as teacher, researcher, and role model. Christman

(1965) saw the CNS not as a separate role but one that increased the clinical depth of already existing functions. However, Christman (1965) and Georgopoulos (1970) added the role of leader/manager to those functions. Oda (1977) described how a CNS can develop her role into action in the clinical area by using three phases identified as clarification, communication, and implementation. During the clarification phase, the CNS identifies specific aspects of her roles, such as practice parameters, and her philosophy of practice. At the same time, the CNS tries to improve her communication and interpersonal skills in order to strengthen direct interactions. Communication is equally important at this role-formative period. Good communication skills and methods can help the CNS in achieving the goals of acceptance and recognition of her value and worth. In her area of practice, once communication and clarification has occurred, the CNS can move on to the implementation of her planned role functions (Oda, 1977).

Professional nursing organizations also have assisted in the development of the CNS role. For example, The American Nurses Association (ANA), in its 1980 social policy statement, defined the characteristics and functions of CNSs, which derive from already described roles. It is helpful for today's CNS to analyze the past struggles to develop the roles of the CNS and to correctly and accurately identify the basic functions they are expected to perform. Role theories that state how people assume roles help in focusing upon the particular skills or functions performed by a CNS. This knowledge clarifies how others' expectations are developed concerning particular CNS functions. Expectations about the CNS by others is called role demand (Hardy, 1978). The CNS's actual behavior, or role enactment, may not reflect these expectations and may also be different from the ideal behavior she should exhibit. Therefore, expectations not realized may lead to conflicting or difficult situations. As a result, the CNS may exhibit role stress from external forces that prevent her from performing her role or from the internal frustrations of trying to enact the role. To dissipate this stress, the CNS may modify her role, thereby creating new or changed role expectations (Padilla & Padilla, 1979).

The changing role expectations of the CNS through recent years is seen in a review of topics listed in the *Nursing Index*. It is interesting to note that although the visibility and acceptance of the CNS is changing, the basic, identified roles for practice have remained relatively constant since their origination. Most of the articles prior to 1980 were written in the late sixties and early seventies and were usually theory or concept articles. For some years, the focus changed to nurse practitioners, as the CNSs faded somewhat from the literature scene when hospital management and administration questioned the need for them. In 1980, articles again began appearing, but this time there were more first-person accounts from working CNSs that reflected the problems and solutions in handling their roles. More patient case studies were being presented as the practitioner role became more important to institutions and society. By 1983, articles revealed the need of the working CNS to more clearly define the roles they were performing and to share that information with administration and other health care personnel. The CNS role has seemed to move from the theoretical planning stage to the implementation stage.

Today, the stage for CNS action seems to be set, as changes in the health care field come at an amazing pace. The *Nursing Index* listed the CNS under "nursing functions" until 1982, but since then the listing has been changed to "nursing roles," signifying a major shift in the acceptance and perception of the CNS. Early CNS articles were mostly from psychiatric and medical-surgical nursing perspectives, but the 1984–1985 literature also reflected the role of the CNS in oncology, gerontology, pediatrics, patient education, and rehabilitation patient care. New areas of CNS nursing are constantly being added, both in and out of the hospital environment.

The future trends for the roles of the CNS seem as broad as the imagination, with the opportunity to make a visible impact on the health care delivery system of the nation. Various new and different autonomous role functions are being reported daily, such as independent health consultants or partners in a health team.

The solutions that today's CNSs devise for their concerns and problems will have an impact on CNS role functioning in the future. These concerns include money earned, third-party reimbursement, power, ability to market their functions and activities, and methods of increasing their visibility to others both in and out of the health care field. Thus, the CNS today may carry the responsibility for the success and even the actual existence of future specialists.

ROLE PROBLEMS

Still one of the major problems facing the CNS today is that of clearly defining a place in the provision of health care. Although the basic functions are not disputed, the method and style of performing those roles are often vague. In the past few years, there have been national conferences for the CNS. It is rare for more than two attendees to identically identify their roles and methods of functioning in their individual institution. Each CNS has her own perception of how best to implement the role, but all agree that one basic function is to provide more complete, more in-depth patient care, both directly and indirectly. Singleton and Nail (1984) discuss many of the problems affecting the roles of the CNS but state that the most essential need is for role clarification in order to have autonomous functioning. The nurse executive may wish to employ advanced practitioners but must also consider the usual problems of inadequate staffing, scheduling, job satisfaction, and the overlapping roles of other health care providers. Where the CNS role can be best used in a bureacratic structure is often unclear to both management and the specialist. The following example tells how role clarification was handled in one institution.

A group of newly hired CNSs in a large teaching hospital faced the role identification problem. There had been no CNSs prior to their being employed at the hospital. After a year of trying to implement the role, people were still asking the (by then dreaded question) "What do you do?" The CNS group met and decided to be their own spokespersons. In order to inform hospital and nursing administration about their functions, they developed a slide tape program defining a CNS by ANA standards and by their job descriptions. They also described the common CNS functions of teaching, research, consultation, and patient care. Then they showed how each CNS adapted those functions to fit the hospital area they served. A humorous handout was developed to accompany the slide show and to give people something to take with them (Figure 2.1). A newly developed CNS philosophy, which directly reflected the hospital and nursing service philosophies, was also prepared for distribution (Figure 2.2). The key hospital personnel were then invited to a luncheon. The slide show and handouts were presented, and there was a short question-and-answer period to fill the remainder of the hour. Many of the administrators were unaware that so much was being done by the CNSs, including contributing to positive public relations outside the hospital. Shortly after the program, the administrators of the hospital district officially adopted the CNS philosophy, and the CNSs were given an official slot on the organizational chart. The question of what roles these CNSs played in their hospital was now clear, which in turn freed them to more effectively perform their functions.

BCHD and the UTHSC now have the services of several types of clinical nurse specialists (CNSs). To obtain maximum benefit from these new models, please read the operating instructions carefully. The choice of model will determine the exact activities and benefits you will derive in providing optimum service and care for your BCHD patients.

PRODUCT DESCRIPTION

A. generic name(s): 1. Clinical nurse specialist.
                      2. Nurse Practitioners.
                      3. Enterostomal therapist.

B. brand name(s):   area   product number

(Individual CNS names—Specialty—telephone number)

PRODUCT FUNCTIONS

The specialists are designed to perform several basic functions that are common to all. These are

1. giving advanced, direct patient care;
2. teaching;
3. consultation; and
4. research.

Each model will adapt the above functions to provide an individual and unique service package to each unit utilizing the CNS. Contact the model that would best help accomplish your patient care. The following is a partial list of the types of functions the CNS can provide

1. direct patient care to high-risk or complicated patients;
2. assess and monitor diabetic, gynecological-oncology, and enterostomal therapy clinic patients;
3. consult on special physical, emotional, or logistic patient care problems;
4. provide nursing grand rounds and formal classroom teaching or direct bedside teaching for professional and paraprofessional health care personnel;
5. provide support to the patient's family;
6. provide discharge planning and patient and family teaching; and
7. develop, implement, or assist in clinical research.

HOW TO ACTIVATE A CLINICAL NURSE SPECIALIST

The CNS will usually be found in the clinical area or at their school. Some models have a shared (joint) appointment between two agencies or departments, such as the UTHSC and Medical Center Hospital. Some models are full time at the hospital. All models are available for patient or other consultations. Some models may be directly contacted at their area of functioning without or with a consult form. Some models may be paged or beeped by the product number. Other methods of contact are formal "request for consult" form, a request written in the physician's order sheet, or by verbal and personal contact. With care and proper handling, the CNS will serve you effectively and efficiently for many years without costly repair or replacement.

Figure 2.1. Introducing: The new, advanced model of the clinical nurse specialist. (*Adapted from handouts prepared by Monica Messer, M.S.N., R.N., Surgical Clinical Nurse Specialist, San Antonio, Texas.*)

PHILOSOPHY

In recognizing that the first priority of the Bexar County Hospital District is to provide the highest quality care to the residents of Bexar County, it is the belief of the district that the clinical nurse specialist (CNS) plays an important and necessary role in the delivery of this care.

DEFINITION

Through advanced education and clinical experience, the CNS is an expert in a specialized area of nursing and serves as a role model of excellence in nursing knowledge and clinical practice.

PURPOSE

The major purposes of the CNS are to

1. Use advanced knowledge and skills to provide and promote high-quality, individualized health care to the residents of Bexar County;
2. participate with academic institutions in the education of health care professionals and paraprofessionals in their specialized areas of expertise;
3. institute and participate in research directed toward the improvement of health care;
4. promote cost-effectiveness through patient and staff education by coordinating and participating in discharge planning and by careful selection and utilization of resources; and
5. consult with others within the health care field to share information and skills for better patient care.

Figure 2.2. Clinical nurse specialist philosophy.

Another ongoing problem facing the CNS role today is that of proving that CNS functions are worthwhile and cost-effective. No other group of health professionals has been scrutinized so closely, with each nursing function weighed for its individual worth. While many CNSs feel constantly pressured, the end result may be extremely beneficial. In today's cost conscious society, the nursing group that has the most opportunity to prove its worth is the CNS group. Evaluation and suggestions for identifying cost-effective functioning is addressed more completely in Chapter 9.

A final point to be considered may not be a problem but deserves serious consideration. This is the legality of the CNS's expanded practice. Nurses in an expanded role expect to be held responsible for their more autonomous professional practice. CNSs are well aware of the need to be accountable for their actions according to their knowledge, experience, and ability to work according to the nursing standards of their areas of specialization. However, they also need to be aware that as they become more visible to the public and other health care professionals, they may become involved with legal situations regardless of their competent practice. Many articles today reflect CNSs personal contact with court action cases. The Regan Report on Nursing Law (April 1983) warns nurse specialists that they are now prime legal targets. This knowledge should not deter the CNSs from practicing but should encourage them to constantly be alert to a potential legal situation.

MAJOR ROLES OF THE CNS

There have been six major roles identified for the CNS.

1. *Practitioner.*   ANA's Social Policy (1980) states that a primary function of the CNS is "direct care of selected patients or clients in any setting, including private practice." The CNS's advanced clinical experience and skills are needed at the bedside. The main reason the CNS would assume direct patient care is so the patient can benefit from her expertise.

2. *Teacher.*   A function that transcends all other roles is teaching because it is constantly being done for patients, families, staff, and students. Since this is considered a major role for the CNS, many nurses are now taking a teaching course during their masters program.

3. *Consultant.*   The ANA Social Policy Statement notes that a major function of a CNS consultant is "interprofessional consultation and collaboration in planning total patient care for the individual and groups of patients" and "intraprofessional consultation with nurse specialists in different clinical areas and nurses in general" (ANA, 1980). The CNS is a human resource in the area of his or her expertise and as such is available to a wide range of patients, health care personnel, and laymen.

4. *Researcher.*   The ANA (1980) states that the CNS should participate "in or conduct research related to the area of specialization". This can be anything from disseminating pertinent research findings in literature among unit nurses to conducting formal research.

5. *Change Agent.*   This is the most difficult role to describe, perform, or understand. It probably is not a role but a result that occurs as the CNS performs other roles. It is usually thought that the change effected by a CNS is one that improves patient care, promotes communication with other health care personnel, and improves the practice of nursing. The only consistent thing about being a change agent is knowing that change is inevitable and perhaps, as a CNS, being able to positively influence its course.

6. *Manager.*   This role usually occurs in institutions that have the CNSs in line rather than staff positions. The management function, although contributing to patient care, usually affects the care indirectly and may take much of the person's efforts, leaving little time for other roles. Some of the activities the CNS performs in this role are hiring and firing, managing budgets, and setting policies and procedures. Leadership is inherent in any CNS role and in line or staff positions but is often more clearly identified in line positions.

Role modeling is a pseudorole. It is not always considered a function. It includes actions that others observe and occurs often unconsciously, as the skilled CNS goes about the business of caring for patients, interacting with other health care personnel, and performing the other mentioned functions.

ROLE DEVELOPMENT IN WORK ENVIRONMENT

The ways in which clinical specialists perform their functions in hospitals have been studied since the early 1950s. In a retrospective study of role development of CNSs based on the work done by Ayers in 1971, several functional phases were identified. These phases are orientation, frustration, implementation, and reassessment (Baker, 1973). Oda (1977) described the development phases as implementation, clarification, and communication. The identified phases are remarkably similar to today's CNS reports, leading one to wonder if the phases are an inherent part of any work experience. If this is true, CNSs just beginning to practice their roles could be oriented to the fact that the stages do happen, which may prevent the severe frustration that leads to burnout, ineffectiveness, and perhaps even the end of the CNS role in that institution. The four stages that will be considered here follow (Baker, 1973):

Stage 1, the orientation stage, is slightly different for each person, depending on past experience. Reactions in this phase range from confusion and anxiety to enthusiasm and evaluation of the role. The "honeymoon syndrome" may be in full force, and reality may not always be correctly assessed. Emotions such as fear, nervousness, optimism, and high hopes sometimes interfere with conceptual knowledge. The new CNS, especially one hired in a staff position, wants to make a good impression on the staff since the implementation of ideas depend on the cooperation of others. The CNS may offer to take an assignment or do a function that is outside her job description in order to make this impression. Most specialists plan to spend a block of time ranging from 3 months to a year to get to know the institution's functioning, the personnel, and the policies.

Stage 2 is the frustration stage. Baker identifies it as a time of crises, when anxiety and depression hit the individual. Most nursing schools teach the theory of change, but knowing intellectually that it may take 2 years to effect a change does not prepare one emotionally to accept it. When 3 months have passed and the CNS sees that she has made no difference in patient care, that people still question her role, that staff still does not utilize her, and that physicians ignore her attempts at collegiality, doubt and despair creep in. She wonders at her own worth and feels that she really may be an impostor who will soon be discovered. If administration is also asking her to justify her worth, the frustration may become unbearable. This is the stage when peer support is absolutely essential.

Stage 3, the implementation stage, is a time of effective intervention. Self-doubts and frustration have been overcome, there has been some progress in accomplishment of goals, and hospital people are starting to recognize and use the CNS's expertise. However, lack of directive structure, lack of self-goals, time management, and evaluation of one's own progress may be stressful at this stage for those who are more used to team work or following the direction of a leader. This leads to the fourth stage.

Stage 4, according to Baker, is the reassessment stage, where role functions are evaluated, reorganized, or further developed. Mutual respect between the CNS and staff hopefully has developed, and administration is supportive of the CNS. New directions and goals are formulated, and the CNS roles become broader in depth as new risks are taken in the work place.

MODEL FOR CYCLIC FUNCTIONING PHASES

If the functions are analyzed in the reality of the working environment, it seems clear that the CNS role phases are cyclic rather than interacting in a circular way and that one does not move completely from one stage to another as experience progresses. Rather, one alternates between effective and ineffective organizational functioning (see Figure 2.3). The CNS's behavior continues along a line of adequate functioning on the job, basically fulfilling one's job description. At times, there are periods of either effective or ineffective functioning. For example, during orientation, the job performance may be adequate although not accomplishing change or improving patient care. The task may be simply to get acquainted and to be completely oriented to every aspect of the job. If that is what the CNS does, she is performing along the adequate line, as expected.

As time progresses and the period of frustration begins, functioning may become ineffective, and the CNS may drop below the adequate line. Then, as she comes out of this stage, she may rise higher above the adequate level than before and perform well, accomplishing goals and becoming more effective. When this level of functioning again becomes smooth and accepted

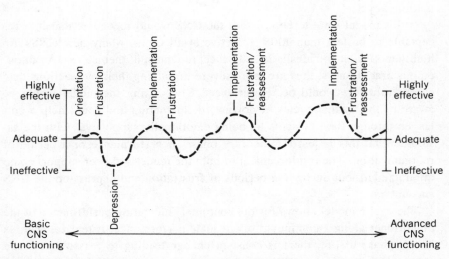

Figure 2.3. Model For cyclic CNS functioning phases: - - - - , nursing function activity.

as normal, the CNS reassesses her goals and devises new ones or attempts new functions. The performance again begins to drop toward the adequate line or below, but not as low as previously. Reassessment and/or reorganization should begin as soon as the CNS notices performance is starting to decrease, although functioning may be still adequate. Another factor that may contribute to a decrease in efficiency is the hospital itself, which is constantly in a state of change. Hospital nursing and administration personnel leave or are replaced, and the CNS may have to prove her worth all over again to new people. This may cause the CNS to modify actions and functions to fit new staffing needs or institutional goals. Again, when change is slow, she may become frustrated and ineffective for a time.

This cyclic period of fluctuation between highly efficient, adequate, and ineffective performance may continue as long as any job continues. The inefficient cycles may be as brief as a few hours or may last for days. As the CNS grows in experience and expertise, she rises higher above the adequate line to become more and more effective over a longer period of time and less and less ineffective for shorter periods of time. Because of the continual change in people and situations, there will always be periods of frustration coupled with minimal performance. The goal of the CNS should be to finally vacillate between periods of high efficiency and adequate functioning as the optimum cycle.

If this model were to be utilized, the CNS would recognize that it is acceptable to be less than 100% effective at all times. Many new CNSs are highly motivated and idealistic and expect too much of themselves. As autonomous practitioners, they are more severe in judging their own actions than other evaluators would be. Experienced CNSs using the model would be aware of the normal cycles of downward fluctuation and could help a colleague through the low spots by being emotionally supportive, with the assurance that this is just a temporary phase of performance or a period of reorganization. The reinforcement of both the model and peer support could minimize burnout during the periods of frustration and depression the CNS encounters.

The cyclic model allows for the continual fluctuating performance of the practitioner along a continuum of adequate performance. It realizes that, as in any phase of life, there is constant change leading to reassessment and reorganization. Most of all, it supports the idea that all workers can expect some down periods in their career but still be productive, valued employers or employees.

FACTORS AFFECTING ROLE FUNCTION

Beginning CNSs, whether experienced or new to the position, begin at the same stage — that of having unclear ideas on what direction they should take to accomplish their functions. Several factors affect the method of functioning in a specialist role. These will be discussed in this section.

The work background of the CNS will determine the method of functioning. Nurses who have a master's degree but little clinical experience differ from nurses with a master's degree who have had extensive clinical experience. Their ability to assess situations and predict clinical problems is better. Experts with experience generally can interact easier with health care personnel and patients, are more skilled technically, and have better, more developed clinical judgment at the beginning of their new work experience (Calkin, 1984). Also, their experience allows them to anticipate and plan instead of being caught by surprise and merely reacting.

Educational preparation will also affect job performance. The CNS must have a master's degree as specified by the ANA. However, not all programs have the same curriculum. One school may include clinical specialization and teaching courses, while another may focus heavily on clinical skills and advanced pathophysiology. Still other schools may teach both areas. Only a few programs include a course in role development.

A job description will affect the CNS's method of functioning. The description will vary from institution to institution. The CNS may be utilized almost exclusively in the teaching role or in management or patient care. Functions and roles will also differ drastically, even if all the same roles are being performed. For example, in one hospital three specialists are employed with identical broad job descriptions. All have similar educational and clinical preparation. However, each performs the roles of teaching, practice, consultation, and research differently, according to the area they serve. The pediatric CNS added a major role by being a strong liaison between nursing and medicine. She actively demonstrated a collegial relationship by being appointed as a faculty member of the pediatric group at the medical school. The oncology CNS organized more patient and family group sessions than the others. She also gave an intensive advanced course to staff nurses to prepare and certify them to give chemotherapy and better care for the cancer patient's total biopsychosocial needs. The diabetes CNS included care both in and out of the hospital. She saw patients at the community level and was involved with public schools and a camp for diabetic children.

Not all facets of CNS functioning in the various roles can be implemented each day or to the same degree in each setting. Differences arise in areas such as critical care, where the patient is in the unit for only a short, intensive time, or in chronic care, where the patient stay is long. If a CNS is involved with orientation, newly hired employees will have different educational needs depending on whether they are experienced or newly graduated and inexperienced.

The immediate needs of the unit served by the CNS may also affect the role functions. At times, direct patient care is needed, such as when technical skills have to be demonstrated to an inexperienced staff or when the patient needs the expertise and knowledge of the CNS. At other times, the consultation role is emphasized because the staff or unit is well developed and able to function without the constant presence of the CNS. At different times, teaching may be more needed. For example, if a new outpatient surgery department is opened in a hospital, the CNS may need to plan and implement a course or series of courses that would prepare staff for the needed new level of care. The research component may be related to the CNS's patient caseload, or other functions, and may be overlapping and ongoing.

Another factor affecting functioning is where the CNS position lies in the organizational structure of the institution. If the position has line rather than staff authority, nursing staff has to tolerate the CNS even if the person is not well liked. The authority that goes with hiring and firing will give this CNS the ability to function differently than those in staff positions. However, it also places the CNS in an evaluative position, which may well be an obstacle. The CNS in a staff position has a different type of authority, which is usually earned over time by using expert knowledge, skills, and the ability to work within the institution to effect change. The CNS with a staff position has to be able to communicate well and to identify areas where her efficiency and knowledge can improve patient care and save money and time for the hospital. For example, a CNS in a staff position working at a county hospital noticed that 75% of the patients on a surgical floor had intravenous (IV) lines for the sole purpose of administering antibiotics postoperatively. The majority of these patients were nonfunded, which meant that supplies used for these patients were paid for by the hospital. The cost of maintaining and administering IV fluids just to ensure patency of the site to administer medications was considerable. The patients did not like the IVs because when they were walking, their lines got caught, infiltrating the IV and making it necessary to restart the IV before the infection control policy time limits.

After noticing and assessing the situation, the CNS suggested changing the IVs to heparin locks in these patients. This was communicated to the head nurse, who supported the idea as a time-saving factor for her nurses. The idea was also communicated in a well-defined memo to the physicians and the nursing administrator, who agreed after seeing the projected cost savings. After the idea was implemented, an audit showed a considerable monetary saving to the hospital. This CNS in a staff position had demonstrated that her items were cost-effective and had saved money for the hospital.

Administrative support drastically affects the CNS's role performance (Edlund, 1983). A CNS who has administrative support can accomplish more in a shorter period of time than one who has no backing, whether official or unofficial. At the same time, the CNS who is able to navigate the bureaucratic waters knowledgeably is better able to accomplish goals within the administrative structure.

The presence of peer support affects the functioning of the CNS. Lack of colleagues with whom to share ideas and derive emotional and professional support can decrease effectiveness in implementing creative and new ideas.

The beginning CNS often has difficulty with time management, which may alter her role performance. This is especially true if the nurse has a dual or joint appointment with two agencies or departments. Since the major roles are fairly well established for clinical specialists, new nurses often feel that they should effectively accomplish all the roles all the time. Nothing could be further from the truth. As stated previously, the roles and functions vary according to the institution's needs at different times. The following short example will demonstrate a variable-function distribution.

Ms. C. S., a pediatric CNS for 4 years, had been working for the past 3 weeks with several young patients and their parents. The staff had consulted Ms. C. S. when two children arrived following a car accident. The children required complex technical care and supportive emotional care for which the staff wanted direction. Once Ms. C. S. was consulted for a patient, she continually followed the child and family through to discharge. The CNS had conducted family sessions and multidisciplinary conferences and had given direct nursing care. Ms. C. S. was at this time mainly performing a direct caregiver role, with minimal consultation and a small amount of teaching for the families. There was no activity on conducting research or in acting as a change agent. However, after the patients had been discharged, Ms. C. S. was called by the Associate Administrator of Nursing to investigate and produce a patient classification system for pediatrics. Ms. C. S. devoted the next several weeks to reviewing the literature, writing up proposals, attending meetings, and finally instituting a pilot project. She was now performing in the change agent role and doing nothing directly as a caregiver or consultant. If she had attempted to continue performing all the role functions, none would have been accomplished completely or well.

The above concept is simple enough to grasp but may be hard to do in reality. If a CNS has a joint appointment, covers many units or departments, or is doing special projects requiring absence from the unit(s) for a period of time, the nurses may begin wondering about her roles, functions, and activities. The old adage "out of sight, out of mind" seems to be the motto. There also may be some professional jealousy toward the CNS for "getting time off" when in fact she may be working many more than 8 hours a day.

There are many strategies that CNSs can use, whether new or experienced, to help them function in their positions (Cooper, 1981) and clarify their role to other health care workers.

One strategy is to be visible. If the CNS is hired to cover many units (such as surgical units plus operating room) or to care for diabetic patients anywhere in the hospital, she must contact each major unit with which she is involved daily. If it is impossible to visit in person, a telephone call should be made. Coffee breaks with the head nurse can be a time for mutual decisions and problem sharing. Other staff, colleagues, or administration must see the CNSs and recognize their presence in the institution. The new CNS may conscientiously avoid the cafeteria or lunchroom or work in her office through break, thinking she must show her ability to work hard. However, not associating with other hospital personnel may cause misinterpretation, leading them to think the CNS is "stand-off" or does not want to associate with them. This opinion can be very detrimental to the CNS in a staff position.

At the beginning of her career, a CNS may choose to help the staff by giving direct patient care when staffing is low. This not only demonstrates the CNS's clinical skill but allows time for staff nurses to feel comfortable with her. However, she should always perform at the advanced level of a CNS and make it clear that her job responsibilities include other functions. Her caseload should gradually adjust to the point where she can actively participate in the other role expectations of the CNS.

Another strategy is to be available to all those who need the services of a CNS or who want to use her for a consultation or as a resource person. If a

CNS is going to be off the main unit or out of the department, a number where she can be reached should be available. If possible, a beeper should be worn. Nothing will dilute job effectiveness more than the nursing staff's inability to contact the CNS if she is needed. Again, there may be special availability problems if the CNS has a joint appointment, at the hospital and at a totally different building, such as a school of nursing.

Specialists who are hired in a staff position have some advantage because they do not evaluate the other workers and so often are trusted with confidences. They can be friendly and helpful to everyone without being seen as threatening. The CNS should learn peoples' names and speak to them on the unit.

Another strategy is to share knowledge and skills as often as possible. This is not the time to be shy and modest. The CNS should communicate ideas, assessments, and suggestions to unit nurses and other health care personnel as often as possible. She should make rounds with the physicians, nurses, and administrators and speak up about opinions or new information. Copies of interesting articles or pertinent clinical research should be made and hung on bulletin boards or put in charts. The CNS should always sign her name on the article, with a "for your information" notice. This is effective for nurses, students, residents, and all other health care personnel and promotes the idea that the CNS is a resource person. The CNS should give large or small and frequent one-on-one inservice programs. She should plan comprehensive educational courses through the Department of Education and Training that all staff caring for a particular population could attend. Finally, the CNS is expected to share knowledge by working on and volunteering for nursing and general hospital committees.

Communication is a major tool. The CNS should formulate in her mind *exactly* what it is she does, so when people ask, the answer can be swift, firm, and without hesitation. It is also imperative to write clear and concise memos, progress notes, nurses notes, and patient care plans. When appropriate, thank you's should be sent to staff and departments. Major meetings between the CNS and administrative personnel should be followed up by a summary of what was discussed, decided, planned, or accomplished. When assigned or identified needed tasks are accomplished, a memo summarizing it should be sent to appropriate people. Scrupulous records should be kept by the CNS on all her activities. She should write self-evaluations and future goals even if there is formal evaluation by the CNS's administrator. Reports should be submitted at specific times, such as monthly, biannually, or yearly, to the appropriate person.

Dress should be congruent to the role of the day. If the CNS is consulting with physicians or working with administration, appropriate business clothes with a lab coat may be worn. If the day's function is to work with students on the unit or give direct patient care, the CNS should wear a uniform. Thus, different people will see the CNS as fitting into their area and better accept her.

There are self-assessment questions the CNS can reflect on in order to judge the effectiveness of her role performance as perceived by others in the clinical area (Cooper, 1981). Some of these thought-provoking questions are:

- Does anyone call for your knowledge and expertise?
- If you have been in the position for a time, are the number of calls the same? Increased? Decreased?
- Do people call you more than once?
- If you are called for consultation, how many of your plans and ideas are put into effect?
- Does staff call you for consultation and then call another CNS for their opinion?
- Do physicians call or write orders for your services?
- Do unit nurses call you for little things? Do they share their personal lives? Do they feel free to complain about problems in the work area?
- Are there units that you cover that never call you?
- Are you appointed to hospital and nursing committees? Made Chair?
- Are you asked to participate or generate research or to write for publication with nurses or physicians?
- Do people in the community know you and request speaking or skill services?

The answers to these questions can help the CNS to identify how others see her. This should enable her to determine if there is a problem in her method of performing her role, to identify strengths and weaknesses, to identify the most frequent role she is asked to perform, or perhaps to further identify and clarify her position as a CNS.

CHANGE AGENT

A chapter about the roles of the CNS would not be complete without a brief discussion of change. As was mentioned previously, many consider that the role of a change agent is really an overlapping function for all CNS activity. The ability to understand and work positively with change will significantly improve the effectiveness of a CNS and increase her value as an employee. Change means to alter something, or make it different, and that is usually what a CNS is thought to do. Understanding theories of change will help the CNS by giving her strategies to work with in implementing change within the work environment.

Three models of change originally described by Chinn (1969) will be discussed here: the systems model, the developmental model, and the model for change. Much of the theory information stems from behavioral science literature in the 1950s and 1960s (Lewin, 1958; Lippitt et al., 1958; Schein & Bennis, 1965; Bennis et al., 1969, 1976). It was often modified and adapted to specific professions, such as nursing (Schlotfeldt & McPhail, 1969). The information is still pertinent and very useful today.

The systems model (Chinn, 1969, p. 299) is often used as a tool for change related to management, organization, and intergroup relations (Schein & Bennis, 1965). It is concerned with rearranging a situation and then regaining a new stability. Successful change in this model depends on how well everything will fit together after the change. The change agent utilizes a problem-solving method of action. She determines the scope, or boundary, of a problem by defining the variables, stress, tension, and conflict surrounding that problem. The conditions that are conducive to achieving change would also be identified. Variables or people that are either resistant to change or ready for change are used in developing a plan of action. The plan is then given a pilot run to see if it is functional and to get feedback. The systems model for effecting change is demonstrated in the following example, in which the CNS identifies a problem, notes the variables, determines the boundaries, and involves the group in the change ideas and decisions. Then a pilot program is run, evaluated, and revised as needed.

A teaching hospital had a large number of student nurses rotating on a nursing unit who had access to the services of a CNS. The hospital had always had students, but recently multiple problems in the unit were adversely affecting patient care. There were overlapping assignments, loss of charges for supplies, physician directions being confused or not done, and multiple medication errors. Staff nurse stress and discontent was increasing with the increase of risks for inadequate patient care. There was decreased learning opportunities for students as staff became less helpful and sharing. The problem could either be structurally altered by stating that the units would not accept students in the future or be dynamically altered by changing the unit policies toward students. The CNS, who was in a staff position, was consulted by the head nurse. After talking with staff and clarifying all the data, the CNS thought that the variables were related to the lack of orientation and direction to students and faculty by the units. The boundaries identified by the head nurse and the CNS were that the students remained in the units and the staff resisted any interaction with the students because they saw them as hinderances and nuisances. The CNS met again with all the nursing staff and asked their input on what they would like to include in a new, unit-specific orientation the CNS would give to students. This would be in addition to the general student orientation by the Department of Education and Training. Using the gathered ideas, the CNS developed an orientation and handout. The CNS oriented the next group of students and helped their teacher become more familiar with the working policies and procedures of the floor. After 3 weeks, the CNS again called a staff meeting to see how the students were doing and if the new orientation had been effective in solving any of the problems. The staff reported that the unit was running much more smoothly, and there were less complaints about the students. The orientation was again revised to include other data and to refine areas of content and procedure. A positive change was being effected using the systems model.

The second method of change is the developmental model (Chinn, p. 305). This model is useful when contemplating change involving person, group, or community interaction. Change in this model is considered natural and inborn in organisms. Problems occur when obstacles hinder the change. Therefore, to be a change agent using this model, one has to diagnose the transitional or critical areas, decide what is stopping change from occurring the way it should, and find ways to remove those obstacles. Several factors have been identified that create obstacles, or resistance to change (Watson, 1969). These can be social factors or individual personality factors. Individual factors include

1. insecurity caused by the unknown role the individual will play with the new change;

2. feelings of self-doubt that the individual can perform as expected in the new situation;

3. habit, or being used to the situation as it was;

4. coping methods of the individual to past change;

5. fear of loss of current job satisfaction, freedom, independence, or power in the organization; and

6. lack of knowledge needed to understand the implications of the planned change.

Social or organizational factors obstructing change may be

1. requiring pressure to institute change with insufficient time for accomplishment,

2. not asking for employee input for change,

3. inflexible plans,

4. a threat to employees' economic or prestige interests,

5. changing areas held to be sacred (ethics, cultures, religion, moral),

6. not considering local or community conditions, and

7. lack of money.

The change agent using the developmental model can also promote growth by preventing obstacles from occurring. These change agents do not impose their own ideas on those involved in the change and are outside the system, such as a consultant from another hospital.

The model for change incorporates elements from both the systems and the developmental models (Chinn, 1969, p. 311). Lewin (1958) defined the terminology and process, which includes unfreezing, changing, and refreezing. The change agent is an insider and an active participant in the change. When a situation is unfrozen, it creates disequilibrium, or breaks a habit. At this point, the direction change will take is still undetermined. When unfreezing occurs, the situation begins changing as participants seek new information and begin rearranging. When the situation again becomes comfortable and stable, refreezing takes place. The choice to change and the direction that will be taken are the responsibility of those involved and are arrived at through a collaborative process. A change agent in this system helps reduce threats and barriers and allows individuals or groups to feel safe and capable of seeking new information. When the group's frame of reference shifts, the new feeling or situation must be confirmed and reinforced as it becomes stable again. A CNS used this model for changing a hospital's way of monitoring glucose levels in diabetics.

The CNS was a diabetic clinical specialist in a community hospital. The patient population served had an extremely high incidence of diabetes that complicated every type of patient's recovery. After an intense study of the situation, attending local and national diabetes meetings, and conferring with researchers and physicians, the CNS determined that monitoring the urine for sugar was not as effective as blood glucose monitoring. Small finger-stick blood-monitoring machines were available that could be used by staff nurses and patients on the units to determine blood glucose levels; the patients could also buy their own machine to take home at discharge. This was a radical new idea for the hospital—to delete urine testing for finger-stick blood testing in the units. To unfreeze the present situation, the personally involved CNS created uneasiness by widely distributing research articles, giving inservice programs, and talking with physicians who supported her point of view. To reduce threats and barriers, she involved representatives from all areas concerned, including doctors, nurses, pharmacy, and lab. She formed a committee to investigate the plan and its implementation and gathered input from as many other people as possible. It became a hospital project as the frame of reference gradually changed from one method to another. The change finally was complete as every nursing unit became educated to the new procedure of finger-stick glucose levels, bought their own machines, and could use them. The lab and pharmacy supported the change. The doctors began ordering only finger-stick monitoring methods. Refreeze had occurred. A major change had been initiated, choreographed, and finally instituted by the CNS. The whole process had taken approximately 2 years.

The CNS can be very effective as a change agent, no matter what role she is involved in. The use of the theory of change cannot always guarantee success but is more likely to effect positive change than unplanned, unrecognized flow of events.

CONCLUSION

The roles of the CNS are valuable and are needed by the patients and the hiring institutions. Teaching, research, patient care, consultation, and management and/or leadership roles all overlap with the function of a change agent. No matter what role is being played or what change is being effected, the CNS is observed and noted by everyone in the health care field. What present and future CNSs do determines the direction of tomorrow's advanced and autonomous nursing practice.

BIBLIOGRAPHY

HEW. (1972). Extending the scope of nursing practice: A report of the secretary's committee to study and extended roles for nurses. Washington, DC: U.S. Government Printing Office, HEW Publication No. (HSM) 73-2037.

American Nurses Association. (1980). Social policy statement. New York: American Nurses Association.

Ayers, R. (1971). The development of the role of the clinical nurse specialist. Phoenix, AZ: City of Hope National Medical Center, Department of Nursing.

Baker, V. (1973). Retrospective explorations in role development. In Reihl, J., & MacVay, J. (Eds.), *The Clinical Nurse Specialist Interpretations*. New York: Appleton-Century-Crofts.

Barrett, J. (1971, July–August). Administration factors in development of new nursing practice roles. *Journal of Nursing Administration*, 1(4), 25–29.

Bennis, K., Benne, K., & Chinn, R. (1969). *The planning of change* (2nd ed.). New York: Holt, Rinehart and Winston.

Bennis, W. G, Benne, K.D., Chinn, R., & Corey, K. E. (1976). *The planning of change* (3rd ed.). New York: Holt, Rinehart and Winston.

Biddle, B., & Thomas, E. (1966). *Role theory: Concepts and research*. New York: Wiley.

Calkin, J. (1984, January). A model for advanced nursing practice. *Journal of Nursing Administration*, **8**, 24–30.

Cooper, D. (1981, February 8). The CNS as a Consultant. Presentation given at a clinical nurse specialist conference. San Francisco, California.

Chinn, R. (1969). The utility of system models and developmental models for practitioners. In Bennis, W. G. (Ed.), *The planning of change: Readings in the applied behavorial sciences* (2nd ed.) (pp. 297–312). New York: Holt, Rinehart and Winston.

Christman, L. (1965). The influence of specialization on the nursing profession. *Nursing Science*, 3(6), 446–453.

Cumulative Index to Nursing Literature. Grandbois, M. (Ed.). Glendale, CA: Seventh-Day Adventist Hospital Association.

Driscol, V. (1973). Liberating nursing practice. The expanded role of the nurse. Browning, E. and E. Lewis. *American Journal of Nursing*.

Edlund, B. J., & Hodges, L. C. (1983, September). Preparing and using the clinical nurse specialist. *Nursing Clinics of North America*, **18**(3), 499–507.

Funk & Wagnall. (1960). *World language dictionary*. Chicago, IL: Encyclopedia Brittanica.

Georgopoulos, B. S., & Christman, L. (1970). The clinical nurse specialist: A role model. *American Journal of Nursing*, **70**, 1030–1039.

Hardy, M. E. (1978). Role stress and role strain. In Hardy, M. E., & Conway, M.E. *Role theory: Perspectives for health Professionals*. New York: Appleton-Century-Crofts.

Lancaster, J., & Lancaster, W. (1982). *The nurse as a change agent*. St. Louis: Mosby.

Lewin, K. (1958). Group decision and Social Change. In MacCoby, E. (Ed.), *Readings in social psychology* (3rd ed.). New York: Holt, Rinehart and Winston.

Linton, R. (1936). *The study of man*. New York: Appleton-Century-Crofts.

Linton, R. (1945). *The cultural background of personality*. New York: Appleton-Century-Crofts.

Lippitt, R., Watson, J., & Westly, B. (1958). *The dynamics of planned change*. New York: Harcourt, Brace and World.

Miller, D. R. (1963). The study of social relationships: Situation, identity, and social interaction. In Koch, S. (Ed.), *Psychology: A study of a science, The process areas, the person, and some applied fields: Their place in psychology and science*. New York: McGraw-Hill.

Oda, D. S. (1977). Specialized role development: A three phase process. *Nursing Outlook*, **25**, 374–377.

Padilla, G. V., & Padilla, G. J. (1979, Winter). Nursing roles to improve patient care. *Nursing Digest*, **6**(4), 1–13.

Peplau, H. (1965, August). Specialization in professional nursing. *Nursing Science*, **2**, 168–295.

Regan, W. (1983, April 11). Nurse specialists: Prime legal targets. Regan Report on Nursing Law, Vol. 23, No. 11.

Schein, E. H., & Bennis, W. G. (1965). *Personal and organizational change through group methods: The laboratory approach*. New York: Wiley.

Schlotfeldt, R., & McPhail, J. (1969, June). An experiment in nursing–Introducing planned change. *American Journal of Nursing,* **69**(6), 1247–1251.

Schramm, C. (1985, March). The clinical nurse specialist. The role in the Or. *AORN Journal*, **41**(3), 579–587.

Sexton, D. (1980, September). Organizational conflict: A creative or destructive force. *Nursing Leadership*, **3**(3), 16–20.

Singleton, E., & Nail, F. (1984, October). Role clarification a prerequisite to autonomy. *Journal of Nursing Administration*, **9**, 17–22.

Sprass, J., & Donoghue, M. (1984, January/February). The future of the oncology clinical nurse specialist. *Oncology Nursing Forum*, **11**(1), 74–78.

Watson, G. (1969). Resistance to change. *The Planning of Change*, (p. 496). New York: Holt, Rinehart and Winston.

CASE STUDY: DEVELOPMENT OF THE CNS ROLE
Evelyn L. Gonzales, M.S.N., R.N.

Ms. N. had a master's degree in nursing, with specialization in critical care. Her graduate program included didactic courses that introduced role development as well as clinical courses that exposed her to practicing CNSs in her chosen field. The clinical courses were her initial introduction to the CNS role.

Upon graduation, she wanted to immediately assume a CNS position in her current place of employment. She was familiar with the hospital system and through the years had been actively involved in projects undertaken in her unit to improve patient care. On many occasions, she had been utilized as an expert resource person. Her qualifications included an educational background that specifically prepared her for a CNS position, and 4 years of clinical nursing experience in critical care. In addition, she had acquired contacts and/or exposure with practicing CNSs over the last year.

Without hesitation, Ms. N. submitted a proposal for a CNS position in critical care to the Director of Nursing (DON) of her institution, a 350-bed community hospital. The DON had read extensively of the benefits of having a CNS in the institution but had not worked with a CNS in the past. Therefore, in considering the creation of the position, input was obtained from nursing and hospital administration. Cost benefit issues and improvement of patient care were the major considerations. The qualifications of Ms. N. were discussed, and after much deliberation, the administration approved the CNS position.

Ms. N. became the first CNS in the institution. She was excited about her position, title, flexible time, and financial remuneration. She had her own office and a secretary. In the organizational structure, Ms. N. was placed directly under the DON and was given the freedom to develop her CNS role. Because of the novelty of her position, the DON and the Staff Development Coordinator were unsure of the orientation that she needed so Ms. N. essentially oriented herself to her new role.

Various sources enabled Ms. N. to develop her job description, including recent knowledge of the CNS role obtained in her master's program and from the literature. She also had samples of CNS job descriptions from other institutions.

Her initial activities were geared toward defining the CNS role and establishing her visibility to various health personnel. The groups she targeted were the critical care staff, including the physicians, allied health personnel, and administration. The reactions that she received to her new role were mixed. Some showed interest, others were curious. There were those who questioned the necessity of a CNS position. She spent a great deal of time trying to define and clarify her role to others while also attempting to assess the system, unit, patient population, and staff practice.

This challenging situation confronted Ms. N. for the first 3 months. She operationalized her job description by identifying tasks that would help her to achieve her goals for the next 6 months. In this process, she integrated concerns expressed by the DON during her job interview. She also took into consideration feedback given by various health team members when she initially introduced her role. Further, she included her own evaluation of the needs of the unit for which she was responsible. To Ms. N.'s amazement, the activities that she wanted to focus on included only education and clinical practice. Her list of planned activities was eight pages long! She went ahead anyway and shared her plans with the DON, who gave her tremendous support and encouragement.

Visibility and accessibility to the critical care staff were goals that Ms. N. wanted to attain. She attended one shift report per day and joined the weekly interdisciplinary team rounds. Through informal discussions with the staff and the head nurses, she identified patient cases that she would be following closely.

Ms. N. decided to take patient assignments during the first few weeks to demonstrate to the staff that she was a competent practitioner. She also made it clear that her job description did not include regular patient assignments. She worked with staff in assisting them to perform complex and unfamiliar procedures. From her perspective, this guidance was needed to enable the staff to become experts. When Ms. N. was told that the staff perceived these activities as spying, she was taken aback. Apparently, the staff felt that the CNS viewed them as incompetent. The staff also perceived the CNS as slowly taking their tasks away from them. Ms. N. then stepped back and reevaluated the situation.

Ms. N. decided to alter her approach with the staff. She concentrated on new staff nurses whom she felt would benefit from her role modeling. She continued to try developing rapport with senior staff nurses by providing positive reinforcement. However, the senior staff nurses continued to see her in a staff nurse position.

To improve the quality of nursing care provided by the staff, she conducted patient care conferences where complex, problematic cases were discussed. The conferences provided the CNS an opportunity to share current theory and research related to nursing diagnosis and interventions. Staff nurses were assisted to present and lead the discussion from which patient care plans were developed. Nurses from different shifts shared the plans, which enhanced communication between nurses. Thus, the staff became more familiar with patients' problems and plans for interventions. This promoted continuity of patient care.

Ms. N. utilized formal inservice programs as well. She developed continuing education courses based on her diagnosis of the educational needs of the staff. In giving lectures and coordinating programs, she involved the staff and other nursing personnel. By recognizing the expertise of others, she gained more cooperation in developing educational activities.

Although many activities kept the CNS occupied, no obvious changes were noted by her, the staff, or the DON. She felt that she had failed the DON's expectations and was losing her support. This internal conflict motivated her to work harder and to strive to do more, which resulted in long work hours and exhaustion with no rewards.

In her self-analysis of her performance, she realized that many of the CNS functional role components overlapped with other personnel. The senior staff nurse provided clinical expertise, the Staff Development Coordinator provided inservice programs, and the head nurse provided consultative services. The CNS role component that was not duplicated by other nursing personnel was research. Ms. N. did not want to focus on research at this time because she felt that more time needed to be devoted to other activities. She continued to keep herself current on research findings related to her field of specialty. Every month, she posted a selected research article in the nurses' station and informally discussed the study with the staff. She utilized these research findings in revising policies and procedures.

In her first 6 months as a CNS, Ms. N. was very busy attempting to develop the role. She had responsibilities for two hospital committees as well as calls for her expertise in other areas. She was beginning to feel pulled in several directions. She was trying hard to fulfill too many expectations. She felt frustrated and no longer knew how to handle the CNS role. Although she felt that she had done her best, she thought she had not accomplished anything that changed the quality of patient care. Therefore, she decided to consult with some of her mentors.

Through networking, she received reassurance and motivation from other CNSs. This helped her readjust to her job and redefine her role as a CNS. She actively participated in professional organizations, particularly the CNS group, and further networked with nurses working in the same specialty. Through interchange of ideas and discussion with practicing CNSs, she realized that her recent experiences were common.

She talked with several CNSs in critical care who had been in the CNS role for varying lengths of time. She found that conferring with experienced CNSs who were stable in their positions was most helpful. They were able to offer diverse strategies in dealing with problems related to the CNS role development in a more objective manner, including how to not overextend herself and how to identify the activities that were most needed at a specific time. Consultation with inexperienced CNSs was helpful in understanding the complexity of the CNS role development. However, it was not very helpful in identifying strategies that helped enhance her success in the CNS role.

Ms. N. had gained additional information about role implementation from her peers. She again reviewed the literature on CNSs but found only a few that described the role, and these were not specific to her needs. Before deciding on plans to further develop her own role, she reevaluated the hospital's environment and her expertise. Again, she identified the needs of the unit, the staff, and the patient and determined the restraining forces in her role development and the resources available to her.

Based on her analysis, she found that one major source of her difficulties was role confusion. She was unsure of how she should function; the people around her did not know how to utilize her. Role boundaries lacked clarity since the CNS role overlapped with other personnel's role. Ms. N. openly discussed her independent and collaborative functions with the staff, head nurse, and staff development coordinator to minimize role conflict. For example, the staff development coordinator would provide inservices on hospitalwide requirements while the CNS would provide inservices specific to critical care.

During the next 6 months, Ms. N. identified her objectives and formulated goals with measurable criteria for each objective. She also identified tasks that facilitated the achievement of her goals. Whenever she had the opportunity, she discussed informally what she did and explained how she could be utilized by the people with whom she worked. In addition, she kept the DON informed about her plans. Because of her better understanding of the CNS role, she was realistic enough not to expect dramatic changes in the quality of patient care in her area. The DON also understood the difficulties in CNS role implementation and was still very supportive. The CNS and DON were aware that while there were no obvious changes in the unit as yet, Ms. N. was working to create change, and it is a slow process.

Instead of evaluating her success based on outcome, she utilized process evaluation. Ms. N. focused on the completion of tasks identified to meet her goals rather than the effect of the task on the quality of patient care. Successful accomplishment of each task that she had identified provided motivation for her to continue with the CNS role.

The patient care conferences and the inservice education programs were well received by the people with whom she worked. She continued to provide positive reinforcement to the staff members who participated in the conferences. The patient care conferences were opened to all members of the interdisciplinary team who were interested in participating. Ms. N.'s role was to facilitate discussion of patient problems and give theoretical rationale for the nursing diagnosis and interventions. Once a month, a topic selected by the staff was provided to all shifts.

As the staff became more familiar with the CNS role, Ms. N. was able to focus on other goals and projects. She planned for time to write articles for journals and to develop research proposals. The staff, head nurse, and Director of Nursing were also included in these projects.

The first 2 years as a CNS had many ups and downs. After the first 2 years, Ms. N. started to feel comfortable with the role functions and activities. She was spending more time with professional organizations and community activities. The recognition that she received from professional involvement reinforced the stability of her job. This resulted in increased respect and support from the staff, other health team members, and the administration.

3

MARKETING YOURSELF AS A CNS

Nancy Girard, M.S.N., R.N.C.S.

Chapter Objectives

At the conclusion of this chapter, the reader will:

1. Discuss marketing strategies for obtaining CNS employment.
2. Recognize the personal and professional qualifications needed to function as a CNS.
3. Identify basic requirements of a resume and job interview.
4. Identify institutional characteristics that might affect potential employment functioning.

Today's health care situation is changing so rapidly that what is fact one day may be obsolete the next. An example is the shortage of good nursing jobs in many areas of the country. Guaranteed employment may no longer exist in many of the nation's hospitals today, so nurses are beginning to become mobile in search of staff nurse positions. Finding employment in advanced nursing jobs, such as clinical specialization, may be doubly difficult. At the same time, specialization is becoming more visible and desirable in many hospitals. One reason is the impact of more and more nurses holding master's degrees who want to work at the patient's bedside. Many hospitals are setting up clinical career ladders and are seeking skilled specialists for the ladder top. Another reason is that there is a closer relationship between schools of nursing and hospitals. Today there are more joint appointments between the two institutions. This instills reality into nursing curricula and answers the needs of hospital administrators who have been requesting better clinically prepared new graduates. There has also been a change in leadership among hospital nursing administrators, including a change in the philosophy of nurses in advanced roles. Nurses who are interested in finding a clinical specialist job may need to market themselves and their ability in today's health care arena. This is a new concept for nurses but may be necessary in order to fulfill career goals. Schools might be wise to include a business course that teaches marketing, sales, and finance in the master's program.

This chapter will give the future CNSs some ideas and tools to compete in the job market and, hopefully, find the employment of their choice. A self-quiz section at the end of the chapter will help the reader identify her own personality characteristics (see Appendix 1).

TRENDS

Many of the trends affecting today's CNS are discussed in other chapters. The activity of the ANA in promoting the CNS by offering certification, forming a council of CNSs, and defining specialization in their social policy statement has greatly increased national awareness and acceptance. Some hospitals are responding to diagnostic-related groups (DRGs) by changing to an all-RN staff. Specialists are being hired to upgrade patient care and fill recognized voids throughout the hospital. The CNS group is becoming larger and more visible. They hold conferences throughout the United States annually, where none were held 6 years ago. They are becoming more sophisticated in marketing, which is promoting the exchange of service of a CNS to those wishing to "purchase" those services. They are also setting up their own businesses, are forming joint practices with physicians, are in charge of nurse-run hospital units, and are becoming more prolific in writing about their experiences. Physicians and other health care providers are becoming aware of CNSs although they may not always fully support them. The territorial battle is just beginning as nurses infringe on the monopoly physicians have held in patient care. A key issue concerning the CNS today is money: determining hospital cost-effectiveness, getting third-party payments for nursing service, or receiving pay for independent, autonomous practice. If the CNS realizes that economics is what makes the health ball go round, she is already ahead of the employment game.

NETWORKING

The student in a master's program who is interested in specialization can begin investigating potential job contacts while still in school. The contacts will be diverse and wide during this time. Faculty with joint appointments would be good contact people. Schools usually have to utilize many different health care institutions in order to provide graduate and undergraduate clinical experience, so the job hunter can talk to students or faculty that have been in those institutions. Physicians are also good contacts. They may be preceptors for graduate students and, by working with nurses who have advanced theory and ability, can see what they have to offer.

Using contacts and professional acquaintances is commonly called *networking*. Networking is important, and there are some guidelines that are helpful to know. The technique of networking seems fairly obvious and an easy thing to do, and some people think "it's who you know that counts!" But it is wise to remember that although using a contact may get a job interview, it is knowledge and skills that obtain and keep the employment. Many job hunters turn off a potential network contact or employer by disobeying common courtesy. The following story demonstrates the misuse of networking.

Jane, a graduate nursing student in a large university school, was talking with some faculty when they mentioned a possible specialist position opening soon at a local hospital. "Who's the nursing director there now?" she asked. Later, Jane called the director and said a professor had referred her. The director granted an interview based on the supposed recommendation of the faculty, whom she knew and respected. When the director decided not to hire Jane, she called the teacher to explain why she had not hired her, much to the unknowing professor's embarrassment. Jane misused her information, and if she had followed correct channels, she may have had a better job opportunity.

Janice Handler (1984), writing in *Savvy* gave seven basic rules for networking:

1. "Make contact based on achievement and stay close at home."

Examples are head nurses or past employers, faculty who have worked closely with a student for more than one short course, and physicians who have witnessed work performance.

2. "When seeking help from people, observe common and uncommon courtesies."

Sally was graduating soon and was job hunting. She asked her favorite teacher for a recommendation, and the teacher gladly provided one for her. Toward the end of the semester, when teaching time was minimal and harried, the student stuck a short handwritten note on the bulletin board outside the teacher's door requesting another written recommendation for an out-of-state hospital. Again the teacher complied, although it compromised her already short time. The third time Sally contacted the teacher, at 3 P.M. on Friday, she sent an even briefer note stating, "I need recommendation for X hospital typed by Monday." The teacher threw the note in the basket and told the student she would not give any more recommendations. The student had not even thanked the teacher verbally for the other two letters! Word spread throughout the faculty, and although the student was a top student, she received no further references from any teacher.

3. "Respect the contact's sense of timing."

If the network contact asks that the potential reference not be contacted until a certain date, the timing should be respected, no matter how anxious or excited the job hunter is.

4. "Be specific about what you want."

Tell the contact person what kind of job is being applied for. Give suggestions about the strengths that could be addressed in a reference letter, including examples of those strengths the contact can remember or relate to.

5. "Do not make unreasonable requests."

Linda won a scholarship from a specialty nursing group during her final school year. She wanted to specialize in that area, and when she attended the award presentation at the group's monthly meeting, she asked several members for referrals. The members were astonished at this "stranger's" request and not only did *not* give her instant references but also wished they could take the award back.

6. "Be appreciative."

Send thank you's or call everyone who has provided references or recommendations. However, do not send a form letter. If a personal note can not be written, it would be better to make a telephone call.

7. "Be helpful to others."

Handler's final suggestion was to emphasize that people should be as willing to help others in seeking positions as others were for them.

MARKETING A CNS

Nurses, as a group, have never had to market themselves. In the past, if there has been an interview connected with being hired, it has been a formality and very brief. Nurses could pick and choose among multiple job offerings in any location in the nation. With the advanced abilities of many nurses seeking employment today, this may not be true. The CNS may have to follow leads and contacts, be assertive, and be able to convince potential employers that they need a CNS. This is not an easy task since nurses are usually self-denying and not used to selling themselves.

The first rule in selling a product, namely the CNS experience and education, is to decide what exactly is being offered. The second rule is to advertise appropriately (Edmunds, 1980). To do this, the CNS must decide exactly what it is she really wants to do. As listed in other chapters, the roles of the CNS are practitioner, teacher, consultant, researcher, change agent, and manager. Identify the role the targeted institution would be most interested in. The only way to determine this is to research the institution well. Never assume that the term *clinical specialist* means the same thing to the institution as to the CNS. Hoffman and Fonteyn (1986) state that knowing the differences between various institutions' needs and identifying the CNS skills that meet those needs is called *market differentiation*. They also identify several benefits the CNS can derive by knowing the different markets:

1. directing the majority of time and effort toward institutions that are of the most interest to her or may be the most receptive of the CNS role;

2. designing educational offerings for the most needed or interested patients, community, or other health care providers;

3. being aware of changes in market needs as soon as they begin;

4. having knowledge of the best time and best method to make a presentation; and

5. having the ability and knowledge needed to gain credibility very quickly.

In reviewing a health care institution for potential employment, the CNS needs to learn as much as possible about it (Hyatt, 1980, p. 119). For example, who are the institution's competitors? What does the local community of health care providers think of the CNS role? Does the hospital already have CNSs that would be willing to talk about employment there? Is there a local ANA council of CNSs that could be joined? If not, are there specialty or other professional organizations who meet locally and could help with needed information about the hospital? After gathering all the data possible about the institution, the CNS must decide what she has to offer.

Perhaps the CNS has identified that the employing institution needs and wants a skilled and experienced practitioner more than the other roles. If this agrees with the CNS's self-goals and interests, the "selling" or "marketing" needs to speak to that area with a heavy emphasis. If all the CNS roles were to be promoted at the same time, the effectiveness of the primary role would be diluted. However, if the preparation for one health care institution does not end with employment, the process of identifying and adapting to another institution's needs should begin again. After determining what role is wanted, the next step in job hunting is the preparation of a resume to submit to the target institution.

RESUME

There are many suggested ways of preparing a resume. One method will be given here, but the reader should be aware that other methods may also be effective. The resume is an introduction to a potential employer. It is still not used extensively among nurses, but if used, it should be done correctly. First impressions are often lasting ones, so make the physical appearance of the resume as perfect as possible. Spend as much time preparing it as would be spent on a major report or project. Remember that there should be an individualized resume for *each* different institution applied to. Do not duplicate one standard copy. The resume should be typed on a high-grade white or light beige paper. There should be no corrected mistakes, and all grammar, spelling, and punctuation should be absolutely perfect. Items should be brief, clear, and concise. Use as few words as possible and leave clean white paper showing around margins and between entries (Edmunds, 1980, p. 43). Often, people applying for positions in large business firms go so far as to have their resumes professionally designed, but there is beginning to be a negative connotation to a "canned" resume. The major categories usually included are experience, education, professional memberships and certification and references. Other items can be added as needed in order to demonstrate CNS ability in the target role being applied for. For example, if the CNS is applying for a nurse researcher position, add thesis, formal research publications, or grants. If the teaching role is the identified area needed for the job, a section can be added that demonstrates writing and verbal communication ability, such as publications, papers presented, inservice programs, or videotapes developed (some authorities recommend a curriculum vita instead of a resume for these positions). A final thought to keep in mind is to be truthful in all areas of a resume. Employers check all the details in today's business world. Figure 3.1 shows a sample resume of a nurse applying for a CNS position in a hospital that is seeking a skilled clinician to improve surgical patient care.

Once the resume is finished, it should be taken or mailed to the potential employer with an introductory cover letter that is also as well done as possible. Do not send a generic, computerized form letter.

THE INTERVIEW

Once the CNS has successfully obtained an interview date, the real work begins. There are several areas for which the CNS should prepare. These include appropriate dress, a portfolio of additional personal data, and information about the interview and setting.

There has been a preponderance of information in recent years about the dress of a business woman or man. The first visual impression of a job applicant, like the resume, is often a lasting one. The grooming aspects should be carefully attended to, from having a neat hairstyle to being sure shoes are polished. Makeup should be carefully applied and not overdone. The clothes should fit the community, the institution, and the person doing the interviewing. One CNS summed up her strategies thus:

Before I obtained my position as Surgical Clinical Specialist at X, a large teaching hospital, I had to interview three different times. The first was with the Nursing Administrator. It was very hot that day and in the South dressing is casual, so I wore a blue silk-cotton blend, shirtwaist style dress. I put a loose, white linen jacket over that. The only jewelry I wore was pearls and my watch and wedding ring. My shoes were white sling pumps. The only item I carried was my leather attache case containing my portfolio. My next interview was with a group consisting of hospital administrators and the board of surgeons — all men. I knew they would also be evaluating how I would represent the hospital at the many community functions the job would require me to attend. For that high level group I chose my only designer suit, an expensive silk blouse, classic pumps, and gold jewelry. I carried nothing, but had business cards with my name, MSN, RN, and home address easily accessible in a pocket. The final meeting was with the staff nurses on the units I would be serving. I did not want to appear stuffy and too formal for them to relate to, so I wore a neat skirt and blouse, low heeled, closed shoes and minimal jewelry. I carried a lab coat with me in case it would be needed. My overall goal was to fit into the company I was interviewing with, and try to have them see the image they wanted for the job. It must have helped. I was hired.

The final word of advice about the proper dress is be yourself and be appropriate.

The second item that needs attention before an interview is the "sales kit," also known as additional information, or a portfolio. The following items are helpful (Hyatt, 1980):

1. *Business cards*. These are not always necessary; however, if you already have cards from your present job, by all means take them along. Some potential employers like to think that the good people they are interviewing do not need a job but may be persuaded to form new alliances for the proper incentive. Cards may help give that impression.

2. *Credentials*. This means anything that might be needed to convince the interviewer that you are qualified for the job. This can include, but is not limited to, copies of documents, such as certification, papers or theses, reprints of articles, awards, continuing education records, media samples, and letters of reference (Edmunds, 1980, p. 46).

The final preparation is for the interview itself. The needed information has been obtained about the institution, but the institution may want more data from the CNS they are considering hiring. The interview situation will be stressful for the CNS, so anything that can be done prior to the interview to reduce the stress will be helpful. If the CNS wants a particular position, that interview should not be the first interview experience. The CNS should go for one or two others first. They do not need to be positions the CNS is very interested in. The role of the CNS as defined earlier is that of an actor. Some people find that it is effective to imagine the interview scene in every conceivable detail and rehearse it thoroughly like an actor. It is also helpful if a friend can play the part of the interviewer. The CNS may make up a list of questions that may be asked and practice the answers until a clear, concise verbal reply can be given for each. Some of the questions may be:

- Why do you want to work here?
- What are your strengths and weaknesses?
- What do you have to offer that our own nurses are not already providing?
- What is your personal philosophy of nursing?
- Would your nursing and social conscience allow you to fully support our for-profit policies?
- Can you work without the authority of a line position?
- Give me some examples of your ability to work independently.
- How can we afford you?

There are also questions that the CNS should have ready to ask the interviewer. They should cover areas that the CNS has decided are important to happiness and the ability to function in a new role. The topics can include the following items:

- Job description.
- Organization structure (chart).
- Administrative support.
- Nursing staff and physician support.
- Presence of other CNS or peers.
- Benefits and salary.
- Mode of nursing delivery.
- Patient groupings (e.g., whether all cancer patients are assigned to one unit or to any unit).
- Orientation.

- Who the CNS will report to and who evaluates her.

As questions and answers are being formulated and practiced, the hopeful CNSs should also be aware of what their body language is saying about them.

When having an interview, the CNS should enter the room confidently but with respect. The CNS should make eye contact. She should introduce herself while offering to shake hands. The handshake should be firm. If possible, she should sit by the side of the desk or interviewer, rather than on the opposite side of the desk, and sit back in the chair. Perching on the edge signifies apprehension and nervousness. The CNS should keep her hands still and not play with pencils, items on the desk, hair or her own fingers. Eye contact should be maintained throughout the interview because staring at a spot over the interviewer's head or looking at a plant while talking can be very distracting for the person being talked to. Negative examples of behavior at an interview are being overfriendly, overconfident, too joking, or superficial. These behaviors usually ensure a continued search. Other attitudes to avoid are being overly compliant and overagreeable. Such persons agree to do all the terrible work situations discussed, answer all the questions before they are asked, and accept too much. If they are offered a job, they may later regret accepting it.

Finally, the knowledgeable interviewee should be aware that there are also topics that are not legally acceptable. These include personal items such as age, children, or intent to have children.

The successful CNS has prepared well, presented well, and passed the hiring regime with flying colors. She has been offered a job, and all that is left to do now is to negotiate the details of the employment.

NEGOTIATIONS OF EMPLOYMENT

A beginning CNS who has little clinical experience and a new master's degree should be realistic about the job benefits and salary offered. However, the experienced nurse with a degree who is job hunting has more to offer and negotiate. It is very difficult to ask for what is desired because the answer may be no, and rejection is hard to take. It takes courage to ask for money, especially if the administrative interviewer was unsure at first about whether they could afford to hire a CNS.

A beginning money figure to request is usually considered to be 10–15%

above the present salary. The CNS should have a realistic view of what the community in general is paying for advanced practitioners. She should read local paper advertisements, call the state nurses' associations, ask colleagues, or talk to those already holding positions. It is helpful to have a low and high figure in mind before the initial interview so there is some flexibility. If the CNS negotiates with the primary goal being money, she should be prepared to refuse or lose employment if the offer is too low. Some examples of financial negotiation statements are:

CNS: "I am sure that if I am offered the position, we can work out a solution."

INTERVIEWER: "An increase in salary after six months can be negotiated at the time of your appointment."

When negotiating for salary, Hyatt (1980, p. 134) states, "If you don't ask for what you are worth, you probably won't get it." However, the health care field is not going to pay the high salaries that occur in business, and the bargaining CNS should keep that in mind. Finally, the CNS should confirm in writing the facts agreed upon during the interview and follow-up.

In business, there are three economic facts to remember (Hyatt, 1980, p. 136):

1. "The economic system is structured so that time and talent have cash values." This agrees with the old proverb that people do not value that which is free.

2. "As you become stronger in your expertise and charge for it accordingly, you enhance your position because you are advertising that you are special and hard to get." The CNS with years of clinical experience and the strong theory base of graduate school is still rare in today's health field. Hospitals are beginning to prize this person.

3. "Set your price realistically, and if it is higher than your interviewer thinks he or she can afford, you have to be willing to be turned down." In general, nursing still is a woman-dominated field. That, plus the economic crunch hitting hospitals, may not allow a salary that is as high as the CNS should get. Other negotiation benefits could be substituted at this point if the interviewer feels strongly that they want the CNS and the CNS wants the job but needs more remuneration.

There are many other benefits that can be considered in negotiation. Some crucial items to consider are financial benefits such as life and disability insurance, paid social security, sick and leave time, relocation expenses, travel funds, and whether the CNS will be working on an hourly salary and punching a time clock or on a set salary. Another thing to consider is office space. Will there be an office for the CNS? Some of the characteristics of space that are highly sought after are location and size, whether it is shared, and if there are windows. Other considerations are if there will be secretarial support for the CNS, and will the hospital pay for certification? Do they support and send the CNS to continuing education outside of the hospital? All these additional benefits can be as important, or more important, than cash in hand. Again, the CNS should be flexible and reasonable with requests.

There are a few final points of negotiation to remember. One is to be sure to negotiate with the correct person. It is not realistic to talk money to the administrator who is doing the interviewing if he or she does not have the power to offer remuneration. Another is to ask clearly, calmly, and directly for what is wanted. Since it is usually difficult for women to ask for money and they are not used to doing so, there are some common mistakes that are made in negotiating. Women apologize about asking, clown or laugh about it, and may even get completely off the track by telling a story about their last employment that is not related to the negotiations. Some examples of negotiating are:

1. CNS: "I am just graduating and want to start a new phase in my career. I'd have to get more than $20,000 or I couldn't accept the job."

Interviewer's thoughts may be: "Don't give me ultimatums. You don't have any job offer yet and are less experienced than I need."

2. CNS: "Well, um, maybe if you thought it sounded reasonable, I could work here for . . . does $20,000 to $25,000 sound too high?"

Interviewer's thoughts: "Boy, is this an example of your self-confidence? If you are unsure what you are worth, how would I know?"

3. CNS: "The CNS position you've described to me sounds very interesting, and there are many responsibilities and duties associated with it. I have accomplished those objectives in my present employment, and I know I can fulfill your needs. However, I'd have to find it worthwhile to leave my present position, which I enjoy. Since I am now aware of your institution's needs,

and I know what my abilities are, I think we could work extremely well together at $25,000."

Interviewer's thoughts: "We can only afford $23,500 for now, but I really like this applicant. Maybe I can give her that big office on the ninth floor and send her to some conferences to make up the difference."

Being aware of effective negotiating guidelines and of verbal and nonverbal communication will put the negotiating CNS ahead of the game.

This chapter has attempted to give the CNS some tools with which to help obtain employment. The final consideration here is the characteristics that will make the new job enjoyable and a success. These characteristics have been mentioned over and over again throughout this book. Four of them are flexibility, creativity, independance, and the ability to take risks. The appendix section following this chapter gives the reader the chance to take some small self-tests to diagnose her own characteristics. These tests are subjective and unscientific and so should be used only as an impetus to internal thought analysis and self-awareness.

BIBLIOGRAPHY

Balint, J., et al. (1983, March/April). Job opportunities for master's prepared nurses. *Nursing Outlook*, **31**(2) 109–114.

Edmunds, M. (1980, June). Developing a marketing portfolio. *Nurse Practitioner*, 941–46.

Hamric, A., & Spross, J. (1983). *The clinical nurse specialist in theory and practice*. New York: Grune & Stratton.

Handler, J. (1984, April). Networking: The rules of the game. *Savvy*, 90–91.

Haserot, P. W. (1985, May/June). Developing a marketing mindset. *The Executive Female*, 26–28.

Hoffman, S. E., & Fonteyn, M. E. (1986, May). The marketing of a clinical nurse specialist. *Nursing Economics*.

Hyatt, C. (1980). Selling when the product is you. *The woman's selling game* (pp. 116–144). New York: Warner Communication.

Johnson, E. P., Wagner, D. H., & Sweeney, J. P. (1984). Identifying the right nurse manager. *Journal of Nursing Administration*, **14**(11), 24–30.

Kotler, P. (1982). *Marketing for nonprofit organizations* (2nd ed.) (p. xiii). Englewood Cliffs, NJ: Prentice-Hall.

LaRocco, S. (1982). Interviewing and selecting staff. *Nursing Management*, **13**(9), 22–24.

Levitt, T. (1981, May–June). Marketing intangible products and product intangibles. *Harvard Business Review*, **59**(3), 94–102.

O'Connor, P. (1984, November–December). *Resumes: Opening the door. Savvy*, **2** (pp. 428–431).

Poteet, G. W. (1984). The employment interview: Avoiding discriminatory questioning. *Journal of Nursing Administration*, **14**(4), 38–42.

Stevens, B. J. (1977). Accountability of the clinical specialist: The administrator's viewpoint. *Nursing Digest*, **5**, 77–79.

Trygstad, J. (1981, March–April). Career milestone: Finding your first job. *Nursing Careers*, **2**(2), 1, 3, 13–14.

Turner, R. H. (1962). Role-taking: Process versus conformity. In Rose, A. M. (Ed.), *Human behavior and social process*. Boston: Houghton Mifflin.

Woodrow, M., & Bell, J. A. (1979). Clinical specialization: Conflict between reality and theory. *Nursing Digest*, **7**, 22–26.

Wooley, A. S. (1983, May–June). How to avoid hard sell and get the job with a better resume. *Nursing Life*, **3**(3), 62–63.

Wright, C. (1984, June 27–July 3). Attending interviews: A positive approach. *Nursing Times*, **80**(26), 44–45.

APPENDIX 1: ARE YOU CREATIVE?

For each question, there can be one of five possible answers. Check the response that most closely resembles your thought. Answer the questions as quickly and truthfully as possible. At the end of the quiz, each answer is given a number value. Add the values to score your creativity.

	Strongly Agree	Agree	Undecided	Disagree	Strongly Disagree
1. I am more interested in a challenging and stimulating job than in salary or power.					
2. All clinical nursing problems can be solved by methodical data collection.					
3. I like to brainstorm and can think up more innovative patient care ideas than others who would be in the session.					
4. If I were not a nurse, I would be an artist.					
5. If I go to the library to look up a subject, I quickly locate my information and leave.					
6. I like to study a management problem from all angles before deciding on the cause and solution.					
7. I can state exactly what is important in my life.					
8. I wonder if the hardness of life is worth-while when I see an elderly patient die.					

(continued)

	Strongly Agree	Agree	Undecided	Disagree	Strongly Disagree
9. I thrive on complex problems in the clinical area.					
10. There is a right way and a wrong way to perform any nursing skill.					

SCORE YOUR CREATIVITY

Mark the number value for each of your answers in the scoring column.

Your Score	Strongly Agree	Agree	Undecided	Disagree	Strongly Disagree	Creativity Scores:
1.	+2	+1	0	−1	−2	16–20 = highly creative
2.	−2	−1	0	+1	+2	
3.	+2	+1	0	−1	−2	11–15 = creative
4.	+2	+1	0	−1	−2	
5.	−2	−1	0	+1	+2	
6.	+2	+1	0	−1	−2	5–10 = average
7.	−2	−1	0	+1	+2	
8.	−2	−1	0	+1	+2	1–4 = oops!
9.	+2	+1	0	−1	−2	
10.	−2	−1	0	+1	+2	

Your Total _____

Clinical creativity can be stimulated by the following:

1. Keep an "idea" folder. Jot flashes of thought and ideas on anything and drop in folder for later reference. (Ideas often flash out of consciousness as fast as they come in.)

2. Question everything! (If you do not improve your creativity, you will have an abundance of clinical research questions.)

3. Think of two or three new ways to do a routine task or procedure, for example, improving shift reports (which usually can use some improving anyway).

4. Do not take yourself too seriously. Laughter helps everyone!

5. Be receptive to new ideas. (You may often get the credit for innovation or for stimulating staff motivation.)

APPENDIX 2:   DO YOU TAKE RISKS?

For each statement or question, there are five possible answers. Check the
answer that best summarizes your feelings about the situation. Answer the
questions as quickly and truthfully as you can. Add the number values of
your answers to get a total and go to the end of this quiz to evaluate your
ability to take risks.

Score as follows:

I would definitely do it	= 5 points				
I might do it	= 4 points				
I do not know	= 3 points				
I probably would not do it	= 2 points				
I would never consider it	= 1 point				

	Would Definitely Do It	Might Do It	Do Not Know	Probably Would Not Do It	Would Never Consider It
1. You have a secure teaching position in a prestigious school of nursing with strong potential to obtain tenure. You are offered the opportunity to have a newly created joint appointment at a hospital as CNS. You would have to give up the tenure slot and lose faculty voting rights. You have no guarantee the hospital will accept a CNS. Would you accept the job?					
2. You have accepted a job as CNS, but you are sharing a small office and storage space with the unit manager. A big office across the hall has become vacant. Another department is negotiating for it. You have unofficial verbal permission to move. Since possession is often not contested, would you move in before getting a more firm commitment in order to beat the other department?					

	Would Definitely Do It	Might Do It	Do Not Know	Probably Would Not Do It	Would Never Consider It
3. Your only chance of getting an innovative patient care change accomplished is to win over a strong, biased surgeon who hates nurses. Would you be brave enough to try and sell the surgeon on your idea?					
4. You are at a national convention with over 500 people present. There is a very prominent nursing leader speaking. You would like to ask a question, but you have to go to a floor microphone. Would you ask your question?					
5. A nurse has told you about her idea for clinical research. You know where you could apply for a grant for that excellent idea. You could then do the research, which would raise your status immeasurably. Would you use her idea?					
6. A colleague friend has invented a needleless syringe that injects solution painlessly. He needs $10,000 to go into production and offers you a percentage of the profits if you will back him. It would take your total savings. Would you back him?					

(continued)

	Would Definitely Do It	Might Do It	Do Not Know	Probably Would Not Do It	Would Never Consider It
7. You are secretly in love with a neighbor who is leaving to join the service. You consider telling him how you feel as you help him pack. Would you?					
8. You are at a hospital board meeting and strongly disagree with the majority of members present. If you speak up, you will anger many influential administrators, and you have been working 6 months to form a positive working relationship with them. Would you speak up?					
9. You observe a technically skilled young resident communicate very inappropriately to patients. Talking to the resident and then to his senior resident has produced no results. You consider going to the resident's faculty physician but know that the whole medical department will be upset at your action. Would you do it?					
10. A patient you are caring for has an incision that looks infected to you. The physician told you it is normal inflammation. Would you make an independent decision as a CNS to culture the wound and then tell the physician about it?					

Each column total =

Add all columns for your score _____

SCORING FOR RISK-TAKERS

45–50 Very high. You may be reckless in your decisions. You might do better as an independent health care entrepreneur than as a CNS. If you score this high, you may want to investigate whether you just like the excitement of high risks or if you really do "look before you leap."

36–44 High. You are very self-confident and ambitious. You probably know that you will be successful as a CNS. You usually are good at generating new ideas, can negotiate well, and are at ease with all those involved with health care.

28–35 Medium. You will do good as a CNS if you have peer support to back and encourage you. You could benefit by learning to feel comfortable with your own ideas to decrease the areas you feel unsure in.

21–27 Low. You are willing to take chances that are fairly safe risks. Concentrate on increasing your self-confidence to act according to your beliefs.

10–20 Very low. Before becoming a CNS, you might want to overcome your fears; otherwise, your chances of being successful and enjoying your job may be slight.

APPENDIX 3:   CAN YOU WORK INDEPENDENTLY?

For each question, there are five possible answers. Check the response that most closely resembles your thoughts. Answer the questions as quickly and truthfully as you can. Scoring is given at the end of the quiz. Add the numbers to give you an idea of your ability to work independently.

	Strongly Agree	Agree	Undecided	Disagree	Strongly Disagree
1. When starting a new job, it would not bother me to have the boss tell me the job description is to "just go out and improve patient care."					
2. I prefer to be chairperson of a committee rather than just a member.					
3. In deciding appropriate patient care, I would always check with the physician and unit head nurse for their input before making a decision.					
4. If there is a diagnosis or treatment I am unfamiliar with, my curiosity leads me to the library to research and learn about it.					
5. I would rather have another health care worker show me how to do a new skill than to practice and learn about it.					
6. I worry that others may see me as too unskilled or lacking in knowledge to be a CNS.					

	Strongly Agree	Agree	Undecided	Disagree	Strongly Disagree
7. It does not make me feel like a failure when a care plan I have spent several hours making is rejected by the unit nurses.					
8. When consulted about a difficult patient care problem, I like to try out solutions that would not occur to others to try.					
9. I know my own weaknesses and attempt to correct them before others have evaluated or discussed them with me.					
10. I am delighted when asked to speak or share my knowledge, opinions, and ideas with others out of and in the hospital.					

(continued)

SCORE YOUR INDEPENDENCE

Mark the number value for each of your answers in the scoring column.

Your Score	Strongly Agree	Agree	Undecided	Disagree	Strongly Disagree
1. _____	+2	+1	0	−1	−2
2. _____	+2	+1	0	−1	−2
3. _____	−2	−1	0	+1	+2
4. _____	+2	+1	0	−1	−2
5. _____	−2	−1	0	+1	+2
6. _____	−2	−1	0	+1	+2
7. _____	+2	+1	0	−1	−2
8. _____	+2	+1	0	−1	−2
9. _____	+2	+1	0	−1	−2
10. _____	+2	+1	0	−1	−2

Your Total _____

16–20 Very high. You can work very independently, without needing approval from anyone except your own standards. You would do very well as a CNS if you do not overstep your legal boundaries and remember to be sensitive to the psychological and managerial needs of others.

11–15 High. You are independent and sensitive. You would do very well as a CNS.

5–10 Average. All other positive considerations included, you should be able to function well as a CNS. You might want to work on decreasing your need for explicit direction.

1–4 Low. Your effectiveness as a CNS might be decreased until you improve your self-concept and ability to plan your own directions in the work place.

APPENDIX 4:   ARE YOU FLEXIBLE?

For each statement or question, there are five possible answers. Check the one that best summarizes your feelings about the situation. Answer the questions as quickly and truthfully as you can. Add the number values of your answers to get a total and go to the end of this quiz to evaluate your flexibility.

Score as follows:

1. It is fine with me — = 5 points
2. Guess I will adjust — = 4 points
3. I do not know — = 3 points
4. It would bother me — = 2 points
5. I would hate it — = 1 point

	Fine with Me	Guess I Will Adjust	I Do Not Know	It Would Bother Me	I Would Hate It
1. You are waiting to give a planned in-service meeting. It has been advertised for 2 weeks, and you have worked hard preparing for it. After waiting 15 minutes, only one nurse has shown up. You have no alternative but to cancel. What are your feelings?					
2. You have been happy in your office for 3 years. The Department of Medicine has just announced they are taking the space for a granted research project. You have no choice but to move. How would you feel?					
3. Your present nursing job involves much orientation and teaching, which you love. Your spouse is being moved, and the only job you can find stresses the practitioner role. What are you thinking?					

(continued)

	Fine with Me	Guess I Will Adjust	I Do Not Know	It Would Bother Me	I Would Hate It
4. You have been working madly all day in order to get off work at 3:30. You have planned to shop for a vacation. As you get ready to leave, the physician calls and asks you to teach a patient to give his own insulin. He also states he has written orders that the patient can be discharged as soon as you see him. What are your thoughts?					
5. The desk is piled high with work. As you settle down to work, you receive three consultation calls and all need tended to immediately. You must skip the desk work, prioritize, and accomplish the requests as soon as possible. How does this affect you?					
6. You enter a room to see a patient and observe a new nurse performing a procedure improperly. You realize you should teach the nurse before caring for the patient, but that will put you behind schedule. How would you do?					
7. A new group of staff nurses are being oriented by you in the routine way. The nurses, however, are very experienced. You need to change your plans and give an expanded and in-depth orientation immediately. What would you think about this?					

	Fine with Me	Guess I Will Adjust	I Do Not Know	It Would Bother Me	I Would Hate It
8. You are teaching technical skills and insist they be done according to the procedure book. One of the nurses states she can do the skill better another way without violating the basic principles. What would you do?					
9. You always play tennis on Wednesday night. It is your only release and outlet. Tonight it is raining and tennis is canceled. How would you feel?					
10. The hospital management states that overtime is not acceptable. Your best nurse has just clocked out 5 minutes late. She has a good excuse. What would you do?					

Each column total

Add all columns for your score _____

SCORING FOR FLEXIBILITY

45–50 So flexible you may sometimes blow in the wind. Better ease up on the relaxation techniques. People might interpret your casualness as wishy-washy if you are not careful.

36–44 Highly flexible. You adapt quickly and well to changes even if you do not always enjoy them. You have broad knowledge and skill bases that allow you to provide extemporaneous teaching and patient care.

26–35   Average flexibility. You are comfortable with your ability to be bothered with unexpected changes and can modify actions to function effectively.

19–25   Some flexibility. In order to decrease the mental strain that goes with a CNS job, you may want to concentrate on why certain things bother you and how you can accept unexpected events more easily.

10–18   Inflexible. You will have to concentrate on not getting so upset with changes or you will get an ulcer.

Cecelia N. Specialist
1849 Education Lane
Health, Ohio 44432
216-654-3210

EXPERIENCE

1981–present	Nursmana General Hospital Head Nurse, Medical-Surgical Unit Supervise a 30-bed unit. Developed policies, audits, procedures, quality controls, and employee evaluations.
1979–1981	Nursmana General Hospital Assistant Head Nurse 30-bed Medical-Surgery Unit Performed care for complex patients and guided care plan formation.
1975–1979	Community General Hospital Staff Nurse 34-bed Medical-Surgery Unit Performed total care for six patients daily that had medical and surgical hospitalizations.

EDUCATION

| Current | University Of Health, Ohio
M.S.N. in progress |
| 1971–1975 | University Of Bowling Red, Ohio
B.S.N. |

PROFESSIONAL MEMBERSHIP/CERTIFICATION

| 1975–current | ANA
Neurosurgical Nurses Association
Infection Control Practitioners |
| 1984 | ANA Medical-Surgical Certification |

REFERENCES   Available on request.

Figure 3.1.   Example of a resume.

4

POWER, POLITICS, AND LEADERSHIP

Shirley W. Menard, M.S.N., R.N.

Chapter Objectives

At the conclusion of this chapter, the reader will:

1. Understand the theoretical basis of power and its relationship to politics and leadership.
2. Describe the types of power a CNS may have and encounter.
3. State the various positions of a CNS in the hospital hierarchy.
4. Discuss the way in which the CNS can become politically active.

"Nurses must develop and use power effectively in order to obtain results in both the nursing profession and the health care system" (Stevens, 1983, p. 3). As the largest group of health care providers in the United States, it would seem that nursing should be the most powerful entity and have the greatest voice (next to health care consumers) in the health care field. This chapter will explore various aspects of power and attempt to look at reasons nurses do or do not have power. It will also address the ways a CNS can use power at all levels.

Claus and Bailey (1977) define *power* as "the ability and willingness to affect the behavior of others." They see power as based on strength and energy that leads to some action that will influence another's behavior (See Figure 4.1). Strength is generally based on a strong self-concept in the person with power. At times we have seen nursing's self-concept weakened by a methodical harrassment of the profession by outside groups who wish to control health care and from within nursing by those who seem afraid to be accountable. In the education of beginning nurses, we must nurture and strengthen that self-concept so that the cycle of powerlessness can be broken.

Kalisch and Kalisch (1982) discuss several theories of power. *Resource* theory relates that power resides with the person who has the greatest resources. Certainly, if one chooses to view this theory in terms of nursing, one can see that since it is physicians and hospitals who hold the resources, it follows that nurses, who hold few resources, would possess little power. A second theory deals with *exchange* and looks at who can offer the most rewards or extract the greatest cost. Once again, when viewed from this standpoint, nursing would come out on the short side of the power. The third theory concerns *decision making* and states that power rests with whoever makes the final decision. Traditionally, medicine has had the last say in all matters pertaining to patient care. The fourth theory is *systems theory* and holds that there is a circular process of interactions between power holders and power subjects. This too can easily be seen in the "doctor–nurse game" as described by Stein (1968). Nurses are the power subjects, and this is reinforced by their interactions with physicians, who are the power holders. In summary, it would appear that nursing does not have power as it pertains to four theoretical perspectives.

Power has many forms, both positive and negative. The nurse who wishes to gain and use power must be aware of these various forms and how they may best be used. Stevens (1983) discusses five forms of power. The first is *exploitative* power, which is destructive. An example of exploitative power

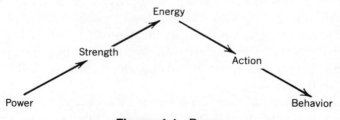

Figure. 4.1. Power.

might be where a nurse forces a child to do something because she is bigger or older than the child. This form should never be used by nursing because it has very negative effects. The second form is *manipulative* power. This indicates power over another and should be used sparingly. Manipulative power can sometimes be seen in the physician–nurse relationship and also in the nurse–patient relationship. When used carefully, it can be a positive force. The third form is *competitive* power, which means power against another. Obviously, this form of power can be good or bad depending on the circumstances. The fourth form deals with the use of power for the benefit of another person and is called *nutrient* power. In the role of advocate, the nurse could use power for the benefit of patients. A final, and the highest, form of power is called *integrative* power. This is power with another. If *all* nursing organizations joined together, just imagine how much power they would have.

Kalisch and Kalisch (1982) present some of the bases of power that allow the person using them to exert power (Figure 4.2). It is extremely important, especially for the CNS, to know these bases and be able to use them intelligently. It is equally important that the CNS recognize when these bases are used by others. The bases include reward, coercion, legitimate power, referent power, and expert power. At this point, it seems appropriate to describe the difference between power and authority. Power is earned while authority is given—usually from administration. The CNS in a line position has authority. The CNS in a line or staff position may have power. One may have authority with no power or power with no authority. In order to use reward or coercion, the CNS must generally be in a line position, that is, be able to hire and fire people. Legitimate power generally also belongs to the line CNS, while the staff CNS has referent power, that is, other people who have power (see Figure 4.3). Both staff and line CNSs have or should have expert power. A discussion of staff versus line position would seem appropriate at this time. Let us look first at the CNS in a line position. The line position

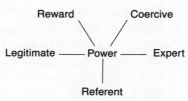

Figure. 4.2. Bases of power.

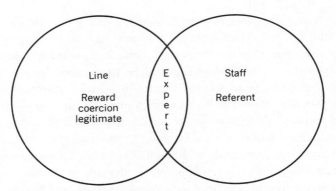

Figure. 4.3. Line CNS power vs. staff CNS power.

held may be that of head nurse, supervisor, or director. With full-time management duties, it would seem difficult to carry on the functions of CNS. A closer look, however, shows that the functions of the CNS may be enhanced by having the legitimate power of the line position. Joel (1985) discusses one line position in use at Rutgers Teaching Nursing Home that appears to work well. The CNS in a staff position has more time to spend in the roles generally associated with clinical specialization but also must expend a great deal of time and energy in wooing the staff to her ideas. It is difficult to recommend one over the other, and this decision must be up to the individual.

In order to use power effectively, it is important to plan the use of that power. The first step in the planned use of power involves leadership. Claus and Bailey (1977, p. 5) define *leadership* as "a set of actions that influence members of a group to move toward goal setting and goal achievement." Leadership must of necessity work from power, for without some degree of power, it is difficult to lead. The CNS must be a good leader in order to make changes, especially if the CNS has no authority to make those changes. Kalisch and Kalisch (1982) state that influence and authority are subdivisions of power. Influence is a willingness of a person to obey someone who lacks formal authority, while authority is a formal right by virtue of the position held. The CNS in a staff position must use influence to make change, while the CNS in a line position has authority to back her up.

There are several influence strategies the CNS can use. These include control of information, expertise, legitimacy, identifying with the leader, rewards and coercion, and manipulation and control of the work environment

(Claus and Bailey, 1977). These can be seen in much the same way as described earlier in the discussion of power. Once again, the CNS must be aware of the various strategies whether she is using them or they are being used on her.

McFarland (1982) looks at some methods by which nurses can use power. One method involves constancy. The nurse is always "there" for the patient. Other caregivers come and go, but nursing is a 24-hour a day presence. It is the nurse who knows the patient best and has the most pertinent information. The patient turns to the nurse for most of his needs, and the physician turns to the nurse for information about how the patient is doing. The physician also has need of the nurse to, as he sees it, care for "his" patient by carrying out physician orders. This constancy gives the nurse a tremendous amount of potential power that is frequently not used appropriately. When a nurse has information regarding the patient or his orders, she turns coy and pretends that the physician has the information. She does not discuss the patient with the physician, thereby taking credit for the knowledge she has. The CNS can demonstrate to other nurses how to share patient or professional information with health care colleagues.

Another way to use power is via expertise. Nursing has grown into a highly complex profession where the generalist is almost extinct. The intensive care nurse has skills much different from the delivery room nurse, yet each person's expertise is equally important. The physician may not be familiar with the technology in a certain area, and therefore the person with power is the nurse—but only if she chooses to exercise that power appropriately. One must also be acutely aware that nursing expertise is different from medical expertise. All too often the nurse looks at nursing as a by product of medicine when each is its own discipline. The nurse with expertise in a given area is not a "junior doctor" but rather should complement the medical care the patient receives. It is important that nursing continue to identify and define nursing practice. The CNS is the ideal person to do this by participating in research activities that broaden the theoretical basis of nursing. The CNS may also help to delineate nursing diagnosis by defining characteristics of specific patient problems. These may then be related to medical diagnoses that may help to identify nursing care costs in relation to diagnostic-related groups (DRGs).

Still another power strategy is the coalition. In nursing, "divide and conquer" has been the rule. Although nursing is the largest group of health care professionals, it has been divided in its approach to problems. The ANA has considered the coalition to be extremely important and has invited other nursing organizations to join together to deal with nursing issues. This kind of cohesiveness can also work well on the local level. The president of the local nursing association can join with the presidents of other nursing groups and in this way begin to present a united front. Coalitions are not limited to nursing, and nurses should remember to join with others whose goals are similar. In the hospital setting, nurses may join with pharmacists to change some aspect of patient medications. Indeed, nurses could align with physicians given the appropriate circumstances.

Use of the media has become extremely important to all who have and/or use power. Traditionally, nurses have not utilized this strategy, yet it is available. One way the CNS can use the media is to provide health information. This can be done as a consultant to the media or as the actual presenter. A group of CNSs in San Antonio, Texas, have developed a slide/tape to show the public how the CNS functions in an expanded role. Nurses have written columns for newspapers and have hosted segments of news programs. Visibility is necessary to gain and retain power.

The legislative power strategy is perhaps the most important and will be discussed later in this chapter. The final strategy for using power (especially in the hospital setting) is the use of collective bargaining or shared governance. Collective bargaining has "union" overtones, but the union may be one made up of all the registered nurses (RNs) in a given institution with no outside help from anyone or it can be any of a number of other unions such as the AFL-CIO. Most nurses object to unions composed of people other than RNs because the issues may not be the same. Collective bargaining using the state professional nursing association is also a possibility; however, some state associations do not do collective bargaining. No matter what union organizational scheme is used, the idea that nurses are joining together to improve patient care is power in action. Depending on her position (line vs. staff), the CNS may or may not join in collective bargaining. She may, however, help nurses to identify problems with delivery of care and the strategies that will best solve those problems. Shared governance has been used in some institutions to give nursing an appropriate place in administrative decisions. The nursing council is made up of elected or appointed representatives from the nursing staff. This council is then responsible for quality of care, including environmental problems and conditions. The council decides on qualifications for practice much as medical staff determines qualifications to practice medicine in the particular institution. Shared governance would seem to be the wave of the future for nursing staffs, but only as they are willing to assume such responsibility. The CNS can help to guide and counsel the staff nurses as they assume this type of leadership role. The CNS can assist staff to utilize the power shared governance brings for the betterment of patient care as well as for staff benefit.

There are rules for using power without abusing it—indeed, the first rule is not to abuse power. Another rule is to never give up one's ethics to play a power game. Power must be used for respectable ends, such as improved patient care. If the nurse cannot or will not follow these simple rules, the power she has will be minimized.

Power in the hospital takes on special significance because 80% of nurses are employed in hospitals. Currently, the administrator of a hospital is usually not a nurse, but Hendricks (1983) recounts that nurses did serve as hospital administrators prior to World War II, but because hospitals became more complex, administration became a separate entity. Power within the hospital hierarchy came to be shared by physicians and administrators, leaving nursing directors with little say.

While some hospitals have placed nursing in a top administrative position (Figure 4.4), it is not unusual to find nursing in an inferior position (See Figure 4.5). It is difficult to bargain for nursing demands when the top positions do not belong to nursing. Storlie (1982) believes that the hierarchy within a hospital promotes powerlessness and that nursing usually is not able to fend off this powerlessness. There are many possible reasons why nursing lacks power within the hospital. The largest is profit. Physicians bring in a great deal of profit because they admit patients. Nurses need to help other professionals see that the major reason a patient is hospitalized is because he needs nursing care. Nurses have only recently begun to substantiate the profit they bring the hospital in many areas. Sovie (1985) reports a study on "costing out" nursing. She compares the cost of care at a cancer hospital and a community hospital in the same city. The Maine legislature has recently passed a law to list nursing on the patient bill. This is a first step toward showing nursing's cost-effectiveness. DRGs may prove to be either a boon or a pitfall for nursing. Nurses must begin to prepare patients for discharge when the patient is admitted. This will require a certain amount of planning and expertise. Additionally, nurses must be willing to say that a patient is not ready for discharge. The CNS may find DRGs to be a major force in convincing administrators that CNSs are not only cost-effective but also money makers for the institution. It is vital that the CNS participate in the collection of data

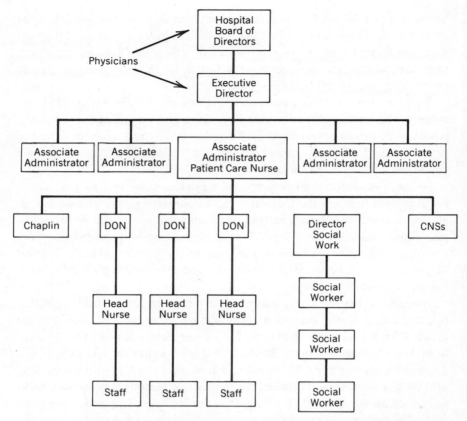

Figure. 4.4. Hospital hierarchy (nurse as administrator).

that may document the savings to the institution. Examples of data may include infection rates, complication rates, and recitivism.

For many years, nursing was part of room and board on the patient bill. Nurses are paid salaries and so are seen only as a cost to the institution. If nurses were able to bill for the patient care they provide, the power of revenue production would be theirs. Additionally, many other departments bill patients for work done by nurses (ECG, lab). As stated previously, physicians admit patients to hospitals, but for a majority of the time patients are in the hospital, it is nursing care (observation, teaching, etc.) that they receive. Although medical orders are also carried out while the patient is hospital-

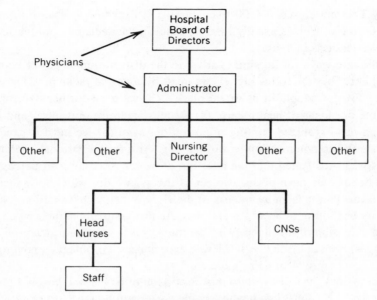

Figure. 4.5. Hospital hierarchy.

ized, they are carried out by the nurse. Also, nurses are not responsible for the high-cost technologies that are in hospitals. It seems strange that physicians are not charged for the space and equipment they use in the hospital. After all, what other profession has their workspace and tools provided free of charge? Hospitals spend millions of dollars on equipment that physicians use for free.

Another major reason for nursing's lack of power may lie within nursing itself, specifically nursing administration. Grissum and Spengler (1976) refer to the "queen bee" syndrome that can be observed in some nursing service directors and head nurses. They have a certain amount of power they use to hold other nurses "in their place." This use, or abuse, of power tends to keep other nurses powerless.

Still a third area has to do with what nursing is or is not. In the past 30 years, many ancillary departments have come into being such as Dietary, Social Service, Respiratory Therapy, and Pharmacy. These areas generally have taken over some of nursing's tasks so that when one of these departments makes a decision, nursing may be affected by that decision. If Respiratory Therapy closes at 6:00 P.M., nursing is expected to absorb the work after 6:00 P.M. Nurses usually have no input in the decision, and the feeling of powerlessness increases.

There are ways for nursing to share in the distribution of power. Sanford (1979) describes the following: (1) we must fill a power vacuum, (2) we must place powerful people in powerful places, (3) we must further develop and promote our ideas of health care, (4) we must exercise our power and ideas through our organized nursing organizations, and (5) we must expand and enhance the communication within nursing. At a recent national conference of CNSs, it was stated that the question of power is a matter of perception. If we believe we have power, we act as though we do, which may increase our power. Power is an awareness of the right of self-determination. Nurses are only beginning to be aware that they are professionals in their own right, not an extension of medicine. We have the power to solve our own problems. A suggestion was made that if nursing experiences a problem enough to discuss it, nursing owns it and should solve it.

Where does the CNS fit into this discussion of power and hospital hierarchies? The CNS must know who has the power and how best to work within the power structure. It is generally easier to do this if one understands the theoretical perspectives of power; however, a few examples of how to approach the gaining and use of power may be helpful.

Situation 1

June Smith, M.S.N., R.N., is a new CNS assigned to a surgical floor. The head nurse seems to be the one who holds the power on the floor, but she is constantly belittling any nurse who comes to her with suggestions on patient care. She regards the CNS as a nuisance with whom she must deal.

QUESTION 1: What are the bases of the head nurse's power?

QUESTION 2: What syndrome is the head nurse displaying?

QUESTION 3: How can June Smith gain power?

Discussion: The head nurse's bases for power are legitimate, reward and coercion. She is displaying the queen bee syndrome, which is an abuse of her power. June will need to carefully form her own base of power. There are two ways to approach this. Both ways lie within June's expertise. If she uses the base of expert power, she can gather documentation and information on improved methods of care, which may boost her power. Another base of power may be referent. The staff nurses may choose to model June's behavior because they respect her expertise.

Situation 2

The CNS on a psychiatric unit is also the head nurse. She believes that patients need to be given some responsibility for their own care if able. The psychiatrist holds a different view and also holds a high position in the hospital hierarchy. In her daily interactions with the psychiatrist, the CNS attempts to slowly introduce the concepts she believes important by way of journal articles and patient care improvements.

QUESTION 1: What theory of power is at work here?

QUESTION 2: What form of power is the CNS using?

QUESTION 3: What power strategy(ies) is the CNS using?

Discussion: The systems theory seems to be at work, with the interactions of the nurse ultimately influencing the behavior of the physician. The nurse is using the manipulative form of power, and her power strategy appears to be the use of expertise to convince the psychiatrist.

POLITICS

"For the health and welfare of the nation and for the future of the nursing profession, nurses must become more involved in the legislative and policy setting processes" (Inouye, 1979, p. 6). The CNS must be a leader in the political arena because it is at the legislative level that change really occurs. Some states have enacted nursing legislation dealing with nurses in the expanded role. This legislation has not come easily, for the legislators must be convinced that these changes are for the betterment of overall health care.

This section is designed to give the CNS a brief overview of political process and then some guidelines for the use of that process. Although this chapter generally speaks to politics at the state level, the information can be extrapolated to local and hospital politics.

Jordan (1983, p. 85) states that "the components of politics are power, competition and conflict." Power has already been discussed. Competition and conflict are the heart of the political game. Kalisch and Kalisch (1982) discuss different types of political conflicts. Vertical conflicts involve people at different levels of power, such as physicians and nurses and horizontal conflicts involve people at the same level, such as within nursing. Kalisch and Kalisch (1982) also discuss three approaches to resolving conflict: capitulation, bargaining, and coercion. The preferred approach should be bargaining; unfortunately, nurses sometimes find it difficult to use bargaining because that usually involves compromise. Nurses must learn to play the political game. The first step in this game involves education for both nurses and legislators. If nurses have no conception of the health care issues, they will be hard put to convince a legislator. The CNS must keep abreast of current issues so that she can educate other nurses as well as legislators. Another step is to overcome apathy. If nurses are educated about the issues but do not register to vote, the battle is lost before it is begun.

Still another step is knowing how the legislature operates and how to get a bill through the maze of state congress (see Figure 4.6). A brief look at this diagram will show why it takes so long to get a bill passed. The state nursing association generally lobbies for those bills important to nursing. The CNS should belong to the professional organization so that she has input on these lobbied bills. It is vital that nurses get to know their local legislators so that the nurses will be able to educate them and get them to carry legislation and support bills crucial to nursing. Personal contact is one thing a legislator will not ignore.

Another area with which every CNS should be intimately familiar is the state nurse practice act. Because licensure is a power of the state, each state has somewhat different practice acts. If you are unfamiliar with the wording of your state nurse practice act, a letter to the Board of Nurse Examiners to request a copy is appropriate. In order to be an expert practitioner, the CNS must know what her boundaries are. Additionally, it is important to know that when the nurse practice act is being amended, any part of it is subject to rapid change, so nursing must be alert to any immediate changes from any source. Many states have difficulty in wording the definition of nursing so as to have less gray areas. In their Social Policy Statement, the ANA (1980) has defined nursing as "the diagnosis and treatment of human responses to actual

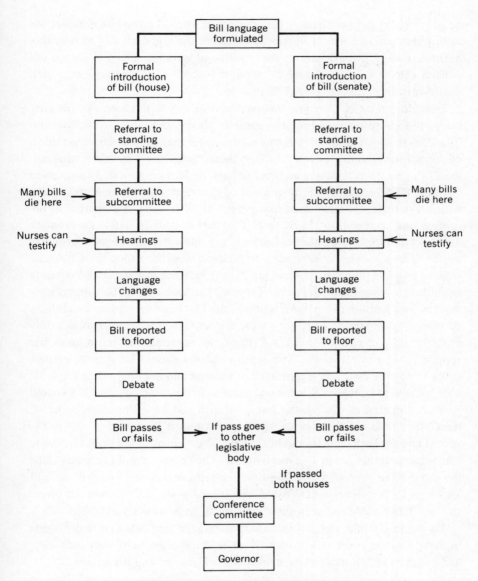

Figure. 4.6. How a bill becomes law.

or potential health problems." This definition could be used as a model for state nurse practice acts if nurses can educate the legislators as to why this definition more fully describes the practice of nursing. The CNS in an expanded role is in an excellent position to lobby for this definition, which would certainly enhance the CNSs practice.

How does the CNS become involved in politics? In the hospital, the first thing to do is to observe how the game is played and who are the players. The CNS must get involved in hospital committee memberships because much of the political gaming is done through these committees. In one institution, the CNS group has a liaison member to each major committee. This helps to keep the CNS in touch with the politics of the institution. In local, state, and national politics, the CNS must first get involved with the local district of the professional association. Each local association usually has a government affairs committee (GAC) that can always use interested members. This committee is responsible for educating legislators. Another group the CNS may want to join is a political action committee (PAC) that is distinct and separate from the professional association. The PAC can lobby for bills, support candidates, and work in campaigns, whereas the GAC cannot support candidates or work in campaigns. In many states, the nursing PACs are seen as a formidable force in politics. Next, a CNS or any nurse should get to know her representatives at all levels. The representatives should be seen at various times to discuss issues of importance to nursing and not only when a crucial vote is about to be taken. When a legislator is first contacted, the CNS should be well prepared to discuss the issues; she should have literature on hand; the CNS should not threaten to work against him if he does not vote as expected and the legislator should not always be expected to see things her way. The important thing is that he has listened. The contact should be maintained throughout the year so that at the time the representative is needed, he will know the CNS well enough to listen. Additionally, the CNS should not forget the legislative aides and secretaries—they can be immensely valuable.

Power, leadership, and politics are important to the CNS who really wants to make an impact on patient care. It takes knowledge, hard work, tenacity, and commitment to make these concepts work for her and for nursing.

BIBLIOGRAPHY

American Nurses Association. (1979). Power: Nursing's challenge for change. New York; American Nurses Association.

American Nurses Association (1980) *Nursing: A Social Policy Statement*. New York: American Nurses Association.

Aiken, L. (1982). The impact of federal health policy on nurses. In Aiken, L. (Ed.), *Nursing in the 80's* (pp. 3–19). New York: American Nurses Association.

Beck, C. (1982, January). The conceptualization of power. In P. Chinn (Ed.), *Advances in Nursing Science*, **4**(2), 1–18.

Bowman, R., & Culpepper, R. (1974, June). Power: Rx for change. *American Journal of Nursing*, **74**(6), 1053–1056.

Claus, K., & Bailey, J. (1977). *Power and influence in health care: A new approach to leadership*. St. Louis: Mosby.

Cleland, V. (1982). Nurses economics and the control of nursing practice. In Aiken L. (Ed.), *Nursing in the 80's*, New York: American Nurses Association.

Crabtree, M. (1979). Effective utilization of clinical specialists within the organizational structure of hospital nursing service. *Nursing Administration Quarterly*, **4**(1), 1–11.

De Santis, G. (1982, January). Power, tactics and the professionalization process. *Nursing and Health Care*, **3**, 14–17, 24.

Diers, D. (1978, January). A different kind of energy: Nurse-power. *Nursing Outlook*, **26**, 51–55.

Grissum, M., & Spengler, C. (1976). *Womanpower and health care*. Boston: Little, Brown.

Hendricks, D. (1983). The power problem. *Nursing Management*, **13**(10), 23–24.

Inouye, D. (1979). Using the legal system to shape nursing practice in power: Nursing's challenge for change. New York: American Nurses Association.

Joel, L. (1985). Preparing clinical specialists for prospective payment. *Patterns in education: The unfolding of nursing*. New York: National League for Nursing.

Jordan, C. (1983). Power of political activity. In Stevens, K. (Ed.), *Power and influence: A source book for nurses*. New York: Wiley.

Kalisch, B. (1978, January). The promise of power. *Nursing Outlook*, **26**, 42–46.

Kallisch, B., & Kalisch, P. (1981, May–June). Communicating clinical nursing issues through the newspaper. *Nursing Research*, **30**(3), 132–138.

Kalisch, B., & Kalisch, P. (1982). *Politics in nursing*. Philadelphia: Lippincott.

Lavatich, T., & Schultheiss, P. (1982). Competition and health manpower issues. In Aiken, L. (Ed.), *Nursing in the 80's*, New York: American Nurses Association.

McFarland, D. (1982). Power as a change strategy. In Lancaster, J., & Lancaster, W. (Eds.), *The nurse as a change agent* (pp. 95–108). St. Louis: Mosby.

Muff, J. (Ed.). (1982). *Socialization, sexism and stereotyping: Woman's issues in nursing* (pp. 359–365). St. Louis: Mosby.

Sanford, N. (1979). Identification and explanation of strategies to develop power for nursing. In *Power: Nursing's challenge for change*, New York: American Nurses Association.

Sovie, M. (1985). Costing out nursing service. *Nursing Management*, **16**(3), 22–28, 32–34, 38, 40, 42.

Stein, L. (1968, January). The doctor–nurse game. *American Journal of Nursing*, **68**, 101–105.

Stevens, K. (Ed.). (1983). *Power and influence: A source book for nurses*. New York: Wiley.

Storlie, F. (1982). Power-getting: A piece of the action. *Nursing Management*, **13**(10), 15–18.

Thomstad, B., Cunningham, N., & Kaplan, B. (1975, July). Changing the rules of the doctor–nurse game. *Nursing Outlook*, **23**, 422–427.

5

THE CNS AS PRACTITIONER

Shirley W. Menard, M.S.N., R.N.

Chapter Objectives

At the conclusion of this chapter, the reader will:

1. Relate the importance of a broad theoretical base to practice.
2. Recognize that the expert use of process is a quality of the CNS.
3. Describe the practical implications of the role of the expert practitioner.

The clinical nurse specialist (CNS) in the role of practitioner is delineated from other nurses in a variety of ways: "Specialization in nursing practice assists in clarifying, revising and strengthening existing practice" (ANA, 1980, p. 22). Because nursing is, above all, a practice profession, it is absolutely essential that the CNS be an expert in her area of practice. The CNS must demonstrate expert clinical judgment. She is able to develop clinical protocols for the care of patients, and she has the ability to manage those patients throughout the course of their illnesses. By means of a high level of problem solving or process, she is able to predict and manage clinical problems before they become unmanageable.

THEORETICAL CONSIDERATIONS

Avant and Walker (1984) discuss the need for nurses to develop conceptual frameworks for their practice. A conceptual framework gives the nurse a basis for organization of care in a logical format. It provides a means of prediction that allows the CNS to formulate interventions based on the need of specific patients and the problems they encounter. Meleis (1985, p. 31) believes that theory guides practice. She states that "theory helps to identify the focus, the means, and the goals of practice." For example, Roy's (1984) conceptual framework tells us that the focus of nursing practice is man. The means (nursing activities) are assessment (of behaviors and factors that influence adaptation level) and intervention by managing the focal, contextual, and residual stimuli. The goal is promotion of adaptation in each adaptive mode (Roy, 1984, pp. 22-23). The CNS who utilizes that particular framework would have a guide for practice.

There are a multitude of theories and conceptual frameworks that a CNS may utilize depending on the specific patient problem. In one instance, systems theory may be selected, and in another instance Orem's self-care framework (1985) is more appropriate. At this point in the development of nursing knowledge, there is no simple theory or framework that can explain all of nursing's phenomena of interest. The ANA's Social Policy Statement (1980, p. 11) states, "The theoretical base for nursing is partially self-generated and partially drawn from other fields: the resulting insights are integrated into a foundation for nursing practice." The CNS who has built upon this foundation adds more depth, clarity, and accountability to her practice.

Nursing process, although basic to the practice of all nurses, provides a framework for developing a high level of clinical judgment. Nursing process consists of essentially four phases, although some authors may use more, each dependent on the others. Nursing process is not static — it must be ongoing or it is of little value. Yura and Walsh (1978, p. 20) describe process as "an orderly, systematic manner of *determining* the client's problems, *making plans* to solve them, *initiating* the plan or assigning others to implement it and *evaluating* the extent to which the plan was effective in resolving the problems identified."

Operational use of the process is broken into four parts: assessment, planning, implementation, and evaluation. The purpose of assessment is to obtain data about the client from a variety of sources. The CNS must be able to utilize all of her senses in the assessment phase in order to determine the needs of the client. When deciding which needs are to be assessed, one can choose from several models. One such model is Maslow's hierarchy of needs (see Figure 5.1). Using this hierarchy, one can assess needs systematically. The ability of the CNS to use a wider perspective of assessment and a more

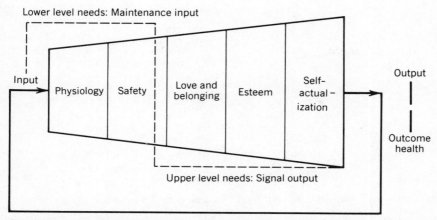

Figure 5.1. Individual As system: hierarchy of Needs. *(From Phipps, W., Long, B., and Woods, N., Medical Surgical Nursing, St. Louis, C. V. Mosby, 1979, p. 21. Used with permission.)*

systematic manner of assessment than is generally expected of nurses appears to add to her credibility as an expert practitioner.

The CNS must be adept in the use of nursing diagnosis. Carpenito's *Handbook of Nursing Diagnosis* (1984) is an excellent resource. The CNS may be in a position to add to the list of acceptable diagnoses because of her expertness in clinical practice. She may be able to offer further etiologic and contributing factors to a diagnosis as well as defining characteristics observed in the individual with that specific diagnosis. Nursing diagnosis is still in its infancy, but with the advent of the National Group for the Classification of Nursing Diagnosis (now called the North American Nursing Diagnosis Association), we have begun to move toward a common language.

It is presupposed that the planning phase of process will include the identification of goals and the writing of an in-depth care plan. The development of care plans based on standards of care and outcome criteria is the mark of the expert clinician. The action phase of process (implementation) should be creative and individual as well as easily adapted to the needs of the patient. The final phase of evaluation completes the cycle and allows one to reassess and readjust the process in terms of patient response.

The use of process may be better illustrated by the utilization of a model (see Figure 5.2). One's view about the nature of process is central to and will

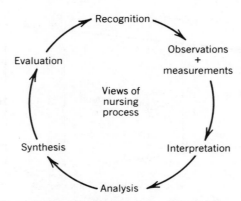

Figure 5.2.   Nursing process: a model for study.

influence the use of process. If one views the process as a vital ongoing flow
of interactions, it follows that all of these interactions will have an impact on
each other. Initially there is a recognition of behaviors. This is influenced by
the broadness of one's theoretical and experiential base. From this basic recognition, observations and measurements are made about changes in the patient state. An interpretation of these changes is made utilizing a theory base.
The nurse then analyzes and synthesizes the information in order to formulate a plan of intervention. Finally, the nurse must evaluate the responses of
the patient to the interventions. This is followed by a recognition of more
behaviors, and so the process goes on.

A new method of looking at process was developed by Menard and Girard
(in preparation). An adaptation of condition diagramming (Russell, 1985)
was utilized to form process diagramming. Condition diagramming is a logical and practical way to synthesize medical information. By adapting this to
nursing process, it is possible to very quickly delineate nursing care problems, interventions, and outcomes (see Figures 5.3a,b).

Practical Considerations

It is all very well to understand the theoretical components of the practitioner
role, but it is equally important that the CNS be able to utilize that theory in
the performance of the practitioner role.

In *Nursing, A Social Policy Statement*, nursing is described as "the diagnosis and treatment of human responses to actual and potential health prob-

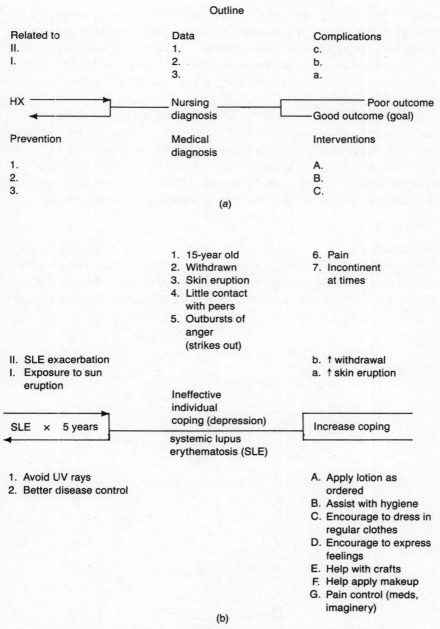

Outline

Related to	Data	Complications
II.	1.	c.
I.	2.	b.
	3.	a.

HX ⟶ Nursing diagnosis ⟶ Poor outcome / Good outcome (goal)

Prevention	Medical diagnosis	Interventions
1.		A.
2.		B.
3.		C.

(a)

Data	
1. 15-year old	6. Pain
2. Withdrawn	7. Incontinent at times
3. Skin eruption	
4. Little contact with peers	
5. Outbursts of anger (strikes out)	

II. SLE exacerbation
I. Exposure to sun eruption

b. ↑ withdrawal
a. ↑ skin eruption

Ineffective individual coping (depression)

SLE × 5 years ⟶ Increase coping

systemic lupus erythematosis (SLE)

1. Avoid UV rays
2. Better disease control

A. Apply lotion as ordered
B. Assist with hygiene
C. Encourage to dress in regular clothes
D. Encourage to express feelings
E. Help with crafts
F. Help apply makeup
G. Pain control (meds, imaginery)

(b)

Figure 5.3. (a) Process diagram. (b) Process diagram applied.

lems" (ANA, 1980, p. 9). The CNS can use this definition as a basis for her practice. It is a simple, yet all-encompassing statement meant to give nursing a substantial foundation on which to build. The CNS must use this definition in a deeper and more complex way than the staff nurse. Although this definition of nursing is grounded in theory, it is also a definition that can easily be applied to practice.

The Social Policy Statement (ANA, 1980) and a model (see Figure 5.4) that looks at practical implications of the role of nursing, may be the framework for expert practice. A brief look at each of the areas from the model will assist the reader in implementing the role of expert practitioner. The theory base is discussed under "Theoretical Considerations" and expert use of process shown by means of two patient situations at the conclusion of the chapter.

Experience

A wide range of experiences is useful to the practitioner for her own growth and because the wider the experience level, the more she is able to share with others. The CNS has had experience in the care of many patients with similar

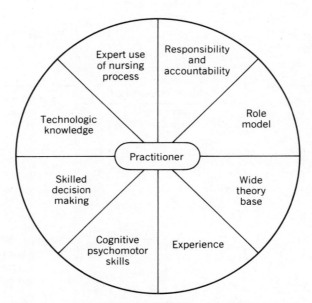

Figure 5.4. The skilled practitioner: a model for practice.

problems. She is able to utilize this experiential base to develop protocols that may be used as the basis for the care of other patients with the same or similar nursing diagnosis. The CNS may develop a protocol for the use of hyperalimentation because she has had many experiences with patients who require hyperalimentation.

Another aspect of experience is the intuitive "flash" that so frequently characterizes the advanced clinical nurse. Intuition is one way of expressing this phenomenon but it may be that it is a rapid and subconscious use of nursing process rather than intuition. Take, for example, the pediatric CNS who during shift report tells the oncoming nurse to carefully monitor the child with meningitis even though his vital signs are normal and he appears to be improving. The CNS has a "feeling" that something is not quite right. Later, the child has a seizure and everyone wonders how the CNS could have foreseen the event. Benner and Wrubel (1982) discuss perceptual awareness which may be similar to intuition. They describe the subtle use of all senses by expert nurses so that they become more quickly aware of changes in the patient. Whatever one chooses to call this special trait of advanced clinical nurses—intuition, process or perception—it is important to remember that experience lays the groundwork for this quality.

Technical Knowledge

As anyone who works in the health care field knows, there is a rapidly expanding array of technical equipment available. The CNS must be aware of the equipment utilized in her specialty area. There must be not only an awareness of equipment but also an understanding of the operational aspects of that equipment. The CNS must be familiar enough with the technology to explain it to others. One's credibility as an "expert" may rapidly diminish if one is unable to explain equipment utilized in one's practice.

As a CNS, it is next to impossible to keep up with everything; however, familiarity with what is currently available in one's specialty is essential. There are several ways to do this. One way is to serve on the product selection committee of the institution. In this way, the CNS will also have input as to which product is best to use.

Another way is to keep in close touch with the sales personnel from various equipment companies—they are always willing to demonstrate equipment. A third way is to read professional journals and informational brochures from various equipment companies. The fourth way for the CNS to maintain expertness in the technological realm is to utilize the specialized equipment on a regular basis. The CNS who is an expert practitioner and accountable for advanced level care must be able to utilize the latest in technology. She should also be the one to institute protocols for patients receiving those technologies. Each of the above methods provides a variety of information that can be used by the CNS.

Cognitive and Psychomotor Skills

For the CNS to function in a believable manner, she must have the necessary psychomotor skills to efficiently perform not only basic skills but also very complex skills. In this area, not only is experience a factor but, of necessity, so is ease with the use of one's hands and mind. The easiest way to maintain the needed proficiency is to set aside time for "hands-on" patient care. Some CNSs prefer to carry their own patient caseload, but this may be difficult to do depending on the time constraints peculiar to each position.

Skilled Decision Maker

All nurses must be able to problem solve their way to a patient care decision. The CNS must be able to do this quickly and with confidence. She needs to be an expert at clinical decision making. That is not to say that the CNS must always have "the right answer" but rather that she must be at ease with the answer given. An illustration of this is the nurse who can comfortably say, "I don't have enough information to make a decision," "I must seek more data," or "I really don't know the answer to that question, but I know where to look." Other staff will look to the CNS for thoughtful, accurate decisions. If the CNS is not able to do this, she will quickly lose the confidence of the staff as well as patients.

Role Model

Role model is a term that is probably one of the most overused in the nurse's language. Although the word is overused, the function is extremely important. It is a case of "do as I do." Staff nurses will look to the action of the expert practitioner for guidance in their own professional life. The staff nurse can easily see a dichotomy if one exists between what the CNS says and does. It is not enough to verbally espouse excellence in care given; the CNS must show via her actions for and interaction with patients that she is capable of providing timely, excellent, and expert care. The staff nurse who sees this kind of excellence in care may be inclined to strive for that same level of care in her daily routine.

The CNS, by virtue of her advanced degree, may also be a role model for nurses and nursing, showing the interplay of education and practice. The CNS is in a perfect position to demonstrate to nurses and other health professionals that an extensive theoretical orientation can successfully be combined with expertness of practice.

Another area where the CNS can be seen as a role model is in interprofessional relationships. The CNS's ability to be seen and respected as a colleague by other health professionals encourages other nurses to assert themselves as contributing members of the health care team. Additionally, the CNS may have a part, via rounds and conferences, in the education of medical students, house staff, and others about the ability of nurses to offer input into patient care decisions. As more health care professionals are exposed to the CNS, old attitudes about nurses and nursing may be eliminated.

Responsibility and Accountability

The final area of discussion is in the degree of responsibility and accountability the CNS as expert practitioner can and should accept. In *Nursing, A Social Pollicy Statement* (ANA, 1980, p. 20), it is stated that

> all nurses are ethically and legally accountable for actions taken in the course of nursing practice as well as for actions delegated by the nurse to others assisting in the delivery of nursing care. Such accountability may be accomplished through the regulatory mechanism of licensure, through criminal and civil laws, through the code of ethics of the profession and through peer evaluation.

The above statement reflects the stand of the ANA on the accountability of each practitioner. How much more is expected of the CNS?

Each CNS must stand ready to accept the more complex responsibilities of her expert practice. The CNS should be accountable enough to her profession and clients to be nationally certified in her specialty area and certified or registered by the Board of Nurse Examiners in the state where she practices if that state has rules and regulations concerning advanced nursing practice. In those states where there are no such rules, the CNS should strive to help the state legislature understand the need for such regulations.

Proof of the expert practice of the CNS should be seen in the documentation of that practice. The CNS may write on nursing progress notes or medical progress notes or both. This documentation is logically formulated and succinctly spells out the problem and its solution. It is also another way of demonstrating one's acceptance of accountability.

Peer evaluation is another way of showing one's accountability . This has proven to be particularly difficult in some areas because many clinical nurse specialists have no peers within their work setting. Without peer and/or self-evaluation, the CNS cannot be certain that goals are being met or that practice is effective. Evaluation of the CNS is discussed in depth in Chapter 9 of this book.

Problem Solving through Process

The expert practitioner should be able to easily utilize process as a method for solving patient care problems. The following clinical situations will illustrate how the CNS may use process.

Clinical Situation 1

Jose was a 37 year-old male with a tracheostomy due to facial and neck injuries. Although all of the proper equipment was available, sterile technique was not fully observed by all personnel. Additionally, the technique of intermittent application of suction pressure was not practiced by all. The amount of suction time varied from 5 to 20 seconds. Little attention was paid to auscultating the chest prior to and following suction, which resulted in too frequent suctioning with its attendant dangers, such as decreased oxygen level, which could precipitate cardiac arrhythmias.

Data

Suction technique varied greatly from procedural norms.

Sterile techniques were not followed by all.

Ausculation was frequently not done to ascertain need to suction.

Care plans contained little information on suctioning.

Sterile equipment was readily available.

Diagnosis

Patient at risk for infection, lower O_2, trauma to tracheal mucosa, and cardiac arrhythmias related to differences in suctioning technique.

Plan

To improve the understanding for and performance of suctioning patients.

Implementation	Rationale
1. The CNS should be a role model for the performance of proper suctioning technique.	"While performing patient care activities with a high degree of proficiency, the CNS (either deliberately or unwittingly) also serves as a behavioral model of expert clinical nursing" (Georgopoulos & Christman, 1970, p. 26).
2. An in-service program on lung assessment skills by the CNS might increase the use of auscultation by staff nurses.	Perhaps some of the staff do not feel comfortable with physical assessment techniques so they just do not use them. If a class is taught on assessment skills, staff will probably be more tuned to using it.
3. Utilize chance or informal conversations as well as formal in-service programs to reinforce use of sterile techniques not only for suctioning but also in other areas.	"The CNS can use incidental conversations or more structured group teaching sessions to improve their knowledge and skills" (Gordon, 1969, p. 36).
4. Directed group discussions may help group to problem solve areas that need improving and ultimately to set goals for quality patient care.	"Collaborative and conscious planning for the improvement of patient care should be an education process for both nursing personnel and the CNS" (Gordon, 1969, p. 35).

Implementation	Rationale
5. Use of care plans to detail individualized suctioning techniques and assessments.	"Kardex info does not automatically ensure optimal nursing care, but such care can't be achieved and maintained consistently or uniformly without some systematic and comprehensive data base" (Georgopoulos & Christman, p. 105).
6. Keep staff notified of research pertaining to suctioning.	"The ultimate responsibility for the dissemination of new knowledge and the development of new nursing methods rests with the CNS. She must be concerned with closing the gap between knowledge and practice — that is, seeing that new nursing knowledge is applied to patient care" (Gordon, 1969, p. 36).

Evaluation

If techniques to improve suctioning are effective, one would expect to see a decrease in tracheostomy and pulmonary infections. Additionally, sterile technique in other procedures should improve. The care plans should be tailored to depict each patient's suctioning needs and technique. Side effects that are a result of improper technique, such as cardiac arrhythmias, should decrease.

Clinical Situation 2

Annie was a 2½-year-old female admitted with a diagnosis of fever and cellulitis of the left lower leg. The social history showed that Annie's mother was married but not to Annie's father. The mother stayed at the bedside as the child would cry whenever the mother left. Additionally, the child would cry and cling to the mother whenever anyone (especially men) approached. While Annie was being bathed, she was noted to have a whitish discharge from the vagina. This was cultured and found to be negative. An assessment of her skin showed a few old bruises, but nothing really significant. Annie was started on IV antibiotics and warm soaks to the area. During the restarting of the IV, Annie lay perfectly still on her back on the table in the treatment room. Her mother was not present. She kept her arm extended and never cried or moved while the IV was being inserted.

Data

2½-year-old female.

Patient lives with mother and stepfather.

Displayed frequent crying and clinging to mother.

Showed extreme fear of personnel, especially men.

Mother appeared to be very protective of child.

Age-inappropriate behavior on painful procedures.

Vaginal discharge, negative results.

Assessment

Potential alteration in parenting; possibility of sexual abuse.

Plan

To evaluate possibility of sexual abuse.

Implementation	Rationale
The CNS may be a role model on the use of consultation with other professionals, i.e., a Social Service consult to ascertain whether this family is known to Child Welfare; consultation with the attending physicians to share assessments.	The use of consultation needs to be learned by the staff nurse. One way to do this is by use of role modeling.
Talk with the child's mother informally to supplement the history already obtained.	The CNS is in an excellent position to counsel with parents and staff due to her advanced skills and listening abilities.
Utilize informal times with staff to help them explore their feelings on abuse.	

Implementation	Rationale
Utilize play with the child to develop trust and to possibly gain further data.	The CNS can demonstrate the many ways in which data may be obtained.

Evaluation

Consultation with Social Service and Child Welfare showed that this family was known to have another sexually abused child.

Consultation with the physicians provided an opportunity to teach the medical students about family dynamics and childhood development.

Conversations with the mother added some concern on her part that her husband might be abusing the child but that she was afraid to confront him.

Utilizing play with a doll, the child undressed the doll and began to explore the doll's body.

The staff was able to verbalize many angry feelings concerning the child. In this way, they were able to work with the mother in a more comfortable manner.

Summary

The role of the expert practitioner is an extremely important one because nursing is an applied science. A wide theory base is essential to the CNS as she influences the practice setting. The CNS is delineated by demonstration of expert clinical judgment, development of protocols, management of complex patient care, and expert use of process. The CNS must be able to relate theory to practice. She may be assisted in developing a framework to do this by use of a model for expert practice that combines role modeling, a wide theory base, experience, skills, decision making, technologic knowledge, use of process, and accountability.

BIBLIOGRAPHY

ANA. (1980). *Nursing: A social policy statement*. New York: American Nurses Association.

Anderson, L. (1970). The clinical nursing expert. In *The Clinical Nurse Specialist* (pp. 180–183). New York: American Journal of Nursing Co.

Aradine, C., & Denyers, M. J. (1973, September/October). Activities and pressures of clinical nurse specialists. *Nursing Research*, **21**(5), 411–418.

Armstrong, M., Dickeson, E., Howe, J., Jones, D., & Snider, M. (Eds.). (1979). *McGraw-Hill handbook of clinical nursing*. (Chapter 1). New York: McGraw-Hill.

Avant, K., & Walker, L. (1984, March/April). The practicing nurse and conceptual frameworks *MCN*, **9**, 87, 88, 90.

Backscheider, J. (1971). The clinical nurse specialist as a practitioner. *Nursing Forum*, **10**(4), 359-377.

Benner, P., & Wrubel, J. (1982, May/June). Skilled clinical knowledge: The value of perceptual awareness. *Nurse Educator*, 11-17.

Bevis, E. O. (1973). *Curriculum building in a nursing-a process*. St. Louis: Mosby.

Blausey, L., Barton, P., & Dicke, R. (1984, January/February). Development of nursing care guidelines: Putting the CNS outcome standard to work. *Oncology Nursing Forum*, **11**(1), 54-58.

Butnarescu, G. (1978). *Perinatal nursing*, Vol. 2, *Reproductive Health*. New York: Wiley.

Campbell, E. (1979). The process of change. In *The Clinical Nurse Specialist* (pp. 89-93). New York: American Journal of Nursing Co.

Carpenito, L. (1983). *Nursing diagnosis: Application to clinical practice*. Philadelphia: Lippincott.

Carpenito, L. (1984). *Handbook of nursing diagnosis*. Philadelphia: Lippincott.

Christman, L. (1971). Nurse-physician communications. In Bullough, B., and Bullough, V. (Eds.), *New dimensions for nurses* (pp. 146-158). New York: Springer.

Daubenmire, M. J., & King, I. (1973). Nursing process models, A systems approach. *Nursing Outlook*, **21**(8), 512-517.

Doyle, M. (1969, September). An environment for the clinical practice of nursing. *Nursing Clinics of North America*, **4**(3), 521-525.

Erickson, F. (1970). Nurse specialist for children. In *The Clincial Nurse Specialist* (pp. 267-273). New York: AJN. American Journal of Nursing Co.

Fawcet, J. (1984). *Analysis and evaluation of conceptual models of nursing*. Philadelphia: Davis.

Gebbie, K. M., & Lavin, M. A. (1974, February). Classifying nursing diagnoses. *American Journal of Nursing*, **74**, 250-253.

Georgopoulos, B., & Christman, L. (1970). The clinical nurse specialist: A role model. In *The clinical nurse specialist*. New York: American Journal of Nursing Co.

Girourard, S. (1978). The role of the CS as change agent: An experiment in preoperative teaching. *International Journal of Nursing Studies*, **15**, 57-65.

Gordon, M. (1969). The clinical specialist as change agent. *Nursing Outlook*, **17**(3), 36-39.

Hazzard, M. E. (1971, September). An overview of systems theory. *Nursing Clinics of North America*, **6**(3), 385-393.

Hellman, C. (1974, March). The making of clinical specialists. *Nursing Outlook*, **22**(3), 165–167.

Holt, F. (1984, October). A theoretical model for clinical specialist practice. *Nursing and Health Care*, **88**, 445–449.

Johnson, D., Wilcox, J., & Moidel, H. (1970). *The clinical specialist*. New York: American Journal of Nursing Co.

Kron, T. (1976). *The management of nursing care: Putting leadership skills to work* (4th ed.). Philadelphia: Saunders.

Little, D. (1970). The nurse specialist. In *The clinical nurse specialist* (pp. 168–179). New York: American Journal of Nursing Co.

Mauksch, I. G. (1975, October). Nursing is coming of age through the practitioner movement: Pro. *American Journal of Nursing*, **75**, 1834–1843.

Meleis, A. (1985). *Theoretical nursing: Development and progress*. Philadelphia: Lippincott.

Menard, S., & Girard, N. *Process diagramming*. In preparation.

Muller, T. G. (1957, January). The clinical specialist in phychiatric nursing. *Nursing Outlook*, **5**, 22–23.

Orem, D. (1985) *Nursing: Concepts of Practice*. New York: McGraw-Hill.

Pearson, L. (1972). The clinical specialist as a role model or motivator. *Nursing Forum*, **11**(1), 71–77.

Phillips, W., Long, B., & Woods, N. (1979). *Medical surgical nursing* (p. 21). St. Louis: Mosby.

Pierce, L. (1972, November/December). Usefulness of a systems approach for problem conceptualization and investigation. *Nursing Research*, **21**(5), 509–512.

Putt, A. (1978). *General systems theory applied to nursing*. Boston: Little, Brown.

Reiter, F. (1971). The nurse clinician. In Bullough, B., and Bullough, V. (Eds.), *New directions for nurses*, (pp. 6–13). New York: Springer.

Rogers, M. (1970). *The theoretical basis of nursing*. Philadelphia: Davis.

Rogers, M. (1972, January). Nursing: To be or not to be. *Nursing Outlook*, **20**(1), 42–46.

Rogers, M. (1975, October). Nursing is coming of age through the practitioner movement: Con. *American Journal of Nursing*, **75**, 1834–1843.

Roy, C. (1984). *Introduction to nursing: An adaptation model*. Englewood, NJ: Prentice-Hall.

Russell, I. (1985). "Condition diagramming": A new approach to teaching clinical integration. *Medical Education*, **19**, 220–225.

Simms, L. (1965, August). The clinical nursing specialist. *Nurisng Outlook*, **13**, 26–28.

Stearly, S. An N., & Crough, V. (1971). Pediatric nurse practitioner. In Bullough, B., and Bullough, V. (Eds.), *New directions for nurses* (pp. 70–76). New York: Springer.

Sutterly, D., & Donnelly, G. (1973). *Perspectives in human development: Nursing throughout the life cycle*. Philadelphia: Lippincott.

Vasey, E. (1979, April). Writing your patient's care plan—efficiently. *Nursing '79*, 67–71.

Vaughan, B. A. (1973, December). Role fusion, diffusion and confusion. *Nursing Clinics of North America*, 8(4), 703–713.

von Bertalanffy, L. (1968). General systems theory: A critical review. In W. Buckley (Ed.), *Modern systems research for the behavioral scientist*. Chicago: Aldine.

Woolley, F. R., Warnick, M., Kane, R., & Dyer, E. (1974). *Problem oriented nursing*. New York: Springer.

Yura, H., & Walsh, M. (1978). *The nursing process: Assessing, planning, implementing and evaluation* (3rd ed.). New York: Appleton-Century-Crofts.

CASE STUDY: THE CNS AS PRACTITIONER
Susan Cooning, M.S., R.N.

For many clinical specialists, the most difficult part of a new CNS role is establishing credibility with the hospital staff. Communicating to co-workers one's areas of expertise is hard to accomplish in a large hospital setting. Nurses are often the harshest critics of a new CNS, whom they perceive as being long on education, and short on "real" nursing skills.

As a new CNS, the greatest difficulty was not in making myself and my specialized skills and knowledge known to nursing staff but in changing roles from an instructor in the Nursing Continuing Education Department to the CNS role. As orientation coordinator, I gained credibility with nursing staff as I precepted new graduates over a 4-week period in various patient care areas. I also learned a great deal about the hospital system and routines as well as learning the names, faces, and personalities of nurses, physicians, respiratory therapists, dietitians, and personnel from other departments. Becoming familiar with the system, management hierarchy, and formal and informal power structures takes time but is of definite advantage to the CNS when defining a new role.

I found that the continuing education role greatly increased my visibility and credibility as a nurse with special expertise throughout the hospital, not just with nurses on the patient care units. I interacted with various department heads and department members such as staff in the laboratory, social services, respiratory therapy, and the pharmacy through my involvement in hospital committees. I often called on various departments to provide "experts" to present their specialized topics through inservices for staff nurses and through orientation for new nurse employees.

The working relationship with nursing management was also enhanced through my continuing education role. I worked closely with head nurses, nursing supervisors, and nursing administration to provide inservice on hospital policies and to provide nursing staff with appropriate continuing education programs. I had a very strong base of support within the nurse management team, which proved invaluable in developing nursing acceptance and utilization of my CNS role.

As a member of the Continuing Education Department, I was viewed not as a part of nursing management but as a clinician. Medical and nursing staff perceived me as a nonthreatening person who could "get things done" within the system. As I attempted to define my CNS skills, this nonthreatening perception of my role persisted.

I also maintained a close working relationship with the Continuing Education Department in my specialist role. Former co-workers included me in their annual planning for educational offerings. By the nature of their roles, the continuing education instructor and the CNS have many common goals. The CNS, while focusing on the patient's clinical problems and teaching needs or when involved in research, is often the first person to identify the nursing staff's knowledge or skill deficits. Maintaining a good working relationship with the Nursing Education Department helps.

Each institution is unique in their utilization of the nurse specialist, but certainly who one reports to and is evaluated by should be established by the CNS early in job negotiations with administration. It was most important to me to be evaluated by nursing and to report to nursing administration. Nurse specialists in other settings are a part of nursing education.

Because of my previous employment within the hospital system, establishing credibility as a "skilled" nurse was not a major hurdle for me in my new CNS role. What proved to be my greatest obstacle was the role evolution from continuing education instructor to CNS. I had to develop a method to "educate" my colleagues, both nurses and physicians, as to what services a CNS could provide. I had to demonstrate how I had grown professionally and personally from "nurse" to "clinical nurse specialist." One way to accomplish this is to develop a brief introductory letter explaining the education and experience background of the CNS, providing a phone number and office location, and specifically describing or listing areas of expertise. This letter can be distributed to all disciplines to further "publicize" and clarify the new CNS role.

The first step I took was to leave the Continuing Education Department. I applied for a newly developed position within Children's Hospital as Nursing Coordinator for the Nutritional Support Service (NSS). The NSS was not only a new concept in our institution but was also new to many hospitals around the country. Our multidisciplinary team included a clinical nutritionist, a pediatric surgeon, a pharmacist, a nurse in the nursing coordinator role, and a pediatric gastroenterologist in the medical coordinator role. Other team members consisted of the three nurses who made up the IV therapy team. As a team member, I worked with the nutritionist to perform individual nutritional assessments and functioned with the physicians in providing recommendations for laboratory monitoring and follow-up on patients receiving parenteral and enteral nutrition. As a CNS, I had responsibilities in providing educational offerings for nurses who would be caring for patients with central lines, receiving enteral nutrition, and receiving central venous hyperalimentation. My CNS responsibilities required developing and writing hospital and nursing policies and procedures related to patients with special nutritional needs. I also was available on a consultant basis when problems in patient care would arise such as feeding intolerances, clotted central lines, or nonocclusive central line dressings. As nurses became more informed and educated in the nursing management of patients with central lines and hyperalimentation, they were better able to "troubleshoot" and problem solve without my assistance. Initially, nurses called on me inappropriately to start difficult IVs. This was not my role, but I responded willingly to any nursing referrals until nurses learned to utilize the IV team or other NSS team members appropriately. Through responding to nursing needs, I was at least visible and able to serve as a role model by contacting appropriate personnel or identifying resources for future use. However, correcting misconceptions about my CNS role was an ongoing process.

Another problem I encountered in my CNS role was *not* being notified by nursing staff when a legitimate patient care problem arose. For example, when a new central line was placed in a patient, hospital policy required automatic referral to the IV team for dressing changes. I had to be very aggressive by making patient rounds on three units and by attending the shift supervisors' report, where this information was typically communicated. Eventually nurses did learn to call on me or the IV team whenever a patient had a new central line.

The second step after accepting the new position with the NSS was to meet with department heads for an information exchange session. The purpose of this formal meeting was twofold: First, to introduce myself in the CNS role and to define services the nutrition team could provide and, second, to identify how each department could utilize the nurse specialist and the NSS to mutual benefit. The problems identified and the goals set in these meetings gave some good directions in defining my CNS role.

Identifying expectations of the CNS by other health care providers gave me some of my first long-range projects in the specialist role. For example, several head nurses expressed a desire to streamline our equipment needs by standardizing the type of IV pump used in our hospital. The biomedical engineer and the directors of purchasing and of central service also voiced a need to standardize equipment for financial and maintenance reasons. This led to a year-long evaluation and comparison of a variety of pumps. In the CNS role, I was responsible for developing criteria for nursing evaluation of pump effectiveness and ease of use and for coordinating trial periods on each unit.

A similar evaluation of the types of IV catheters used in our hospital also resulted from the formal interviews I conducted with different departments. The most valuable thing I learned from this process is that once you ask a department for input, you have to be prepared to follow through and provide feedback.

I have found that certain strategies that helped me establish my CNS role the first time have served me well in my role in a different institution. Identifying and establishing a base of support within nursing, whether it be through nursing management members, other nurse specialists, or nursing continuing education staff, is key. The support group can offer valuable encouragement as well as constructive criticism of the CNS role. A methodical, organized method of orientation to the hospital system is important. This may be adequately provided by the institution or it may require self-initiation. Defining your CNS role and responsibilities with key personnel and asking for their perceptions in a formal way can be crucial. These meetings increase the specialist's visibility and can be the beginning of establishing professional credibility. Becoming involved in hospital and nursing committees can help in developing credibility and in establishing good liaisons with many disciplines.

Many nurses graduating from their master's degree program, struggling to implement their CNS role for the first time, identify a "credibility gap" between education and advanced nursing practice. Some nurses with graduate degrees feel their educational program did not prepare them for the nurse specialist role. A course in role development is essential. In my graduate program, faculty were either "master educators" or "master researchers," but few were "master clinicians." I had to closely examine my career goals and my expectations of graduate education before I selected and enrolled in my master's program. I found that some programs provide more emphasis for students on developing clinical expertise as practitioners where other programs assume that the graduate nursing student brings with them a certain level of clinical proficiency. These latter programs focus more on nursing research, management, and educator roles of the nurse specialist.

Although much of my learning of my clinical specialty in nutrition did not occur in graduate school, advanced education aided me greatly in my specialist role of marketing, implementing, and evaluating a new service. Advanced education also provided me with the management tools and leadership skills to manage and evaluate individual nurses on the IV team. More in-depth knowledge of teaching and learning principles and instructional and evaluation techniques aided me in developing better educational programs for staff as well as for developing teaching tools for patients and their families. My education better prepared me to interpret and apply research findings to a greater depth in clinical practice. Many clinical questions arise in a new specialty area such as nutrition support, and graduate education prepared me to develop and define research proposals and to implement research methods to answer those questions.

One thing I have learned to accept is that being a "specialist" in an area does not mean you have all the answers. There are always new patient situations or conditions that send me back to the reference books, the latest research findings, or to other experts. Lifelong learning and recognition of one's limitations is also a part of the CNS role.

6

THE CNS AS TEACHER

Julie S. Meyer, M.S.N., R.N.

Chapter Objectives

At the conclusion of this chapter, the reader will:

1. Discuss teaching–learning theory as applied in the health care setting.
2. Recognize the characteristics of an effective teacher.
2. Discuss practical implications for the CNS in the role of teacher.

Teaching is well recognized as an important responsibility for *all* professional nurses. It has been said by Banta (1979) that "nurses must recognize that their primary role as health professionals is that of educator. Only by education are we likely to make inroads in changing behaviors." For the clinical nurse specialist (CNS) this role has special meaning and holds much excitement and challenge. Because of expertise in a particular clinical field and in health teaching and health assessment, the CNS is the most logical person to provide health teaching and health maintenance aspects of care (Draye & Pesznecker, 1980).

While teaching is a separate role, it cannot be separated from the other CNS roles (see Figure 6.1). For example, as an expert practitioner giving direct patient care, the CNS silently teaches other nurses through role modeling. In the consultant role, does not learning occur when the CNS provides specialized information and experience to help others problem solve? And as a researcher, the CNS scientifically gathers existing information to provide

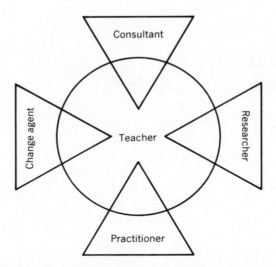

Figure 6.1.   The teacher role is part of all CNS roles.

new knowledge for others. All of these activities involve the teaching–learning process, so the CNS cannot escape the teacher role for more
favored activities. The opportunities for the CNS to teach about health and
illness are limitless. The goal then should be to become a truly effective
educator utilizing teaching–learning theory and principles as a basis.

THEORETICAL PERSPECTIVES

There are many theories that attempt to explain how learning occurs, and
although it is not the purpose of this chapter to discuss these educational
theories in detail, it is useful to take a brief look at two general categories of
learning theory as described by Bigge (1971), behaviorist theory, and Gestalt
field theory.

The behaviorist category includes all the behavioristic stimulus–response
conditioning theories. According to the behaviorists, learning is defined as a
change in behavior that occurs as a response to internal or external environmental stimuli. The Gestalt field theorists define learning as "a process of
gaining or changing insights, outlooks, or thought patterns" (Bigge, 1971, p.
13).

From these definitions, one can see very distinct differences. Even the terminology used by these two groups of theorists in describing the learning process clearly emphasizes the difference in orientation.

Behaviorist Terms	Gestalt Field Terms
Organism	Person
Physical or biological environment	Psychological environment
Action or reaction	Interaction

The goal, then, of the behaviorist teacher is to make a significant change in the learners' *behavior*, whereas the goal of the Gestalt-field-oriented teacher is to help the learners change their *understanding* of situations and problems that are significant (Bigge, 1971).

Because of the complexity and the unending variety of teaching–learning situations in the health care setting, it is obvious that strict exclusive adherence to either of these theories would be very limiting and at times inappropriate. For example, a diabetic patient may not be able to, or may not be interested in, understanding the pathophysiology of hypoglycemia, but he can be taught to memorize the symptoms and respond to them despite lack of understanding. Since it is the patient's correct response that is desired in this situation, the behaviorist approach to teaching is probably adequate. This same diabetic patient, however, may need a different approach when he continues to be noncompliant about following his diet. In order to change his eating habits, he may need help in gaining understanding and insight into the relationship of food intake to blood glucose levels and to long-term complications. He may also need assistance in understanding his noncompliant behavior. A Gestalt field approach, therefore, would be more appropriate in helping the patient learn these relationships.

Because of the obvious advantages and disadvantages of both theories, it is important for the CNS to draw from both theoretical bases when planning and implementing teaching activities.

Learning Principles

While some knowledge of learning theories may be helpful, it is more practical to place emphasis on the fundamental principles of learning to assist in providing effective education about health and illness. Of the 12 learning principles described by Margaret Pohl (1973), 5 are particularly pertinent (p. 24). These principles apply across the board, whether one is teaching patients and families, staff nurses, or students.

1. *Physical and Mental Readiness Are Necessary for Learning.* Assessment of readiness to learn is extremely important, especially in the hospital setting, where anxiety levels are usually high for both patients and staff. It goes without saying that if the person is not "ready" to learn, learning will not occur regardless of how "ready" the teacher is to teach. Assessing readiness can prevent wasted time and frustration for the CNS and can also prevent increased stress for the learner.

When a patient is first admitted to the hospital, the nurse collects general information that not only identifies the possible learning needs but also gives clues to whether the patient is *ready* or *able* to learn. For example, what is the diagnosis? How sick is the patient? What is the level of pain or discomfort? What is the mental status – alert? depressed? anxious? diminished? What is the age, ethnic or cultural background, socioeconomic level? The answers to all of these questions will affect readiness to learn.

EXAMPLE 1. An inservice program was planned for the night shift at 7:15 A.M. This was usually a good time, and the nurses were paid for the time. However, this particular night they were short staffed and had three emergency admissions and a high number of very sick patients. The staff was exhausted, but the inservice program was conducted as scheduled. Were these nurses mentally ready to learn? Probably not.

A better approach would have been to compliment the staff on their hard work, cancel the inservice program, and reschedule it for the next evening at 10:30 P.M. when the staff was mentally fresh – even though it might be less convenient for the instructor.

EXAMPLE 2. Mr. Smith received multiple injuries in an automobile accident, including a fractured tibia. He needs to learn crutch walking, but he is extremely weak due to blood loss and prolonged bed rest. He may not be physically ready to learn this skill even though he is mentally prepared to do so.

These two examples show how fruitless it is to try to teach if the student is not ready to learn.

2. *An Individual Must Be Motivated To Learn.*   Motivation is possibly the single most important factor in learning. It is an internal force that makes an individual take action to do something. It can come from an internal stimulus or an external stimulus, and it can be a very short, impulsive action or a long-term, sustained drive. It is important to remember that motivation comes from *inside* the individual and cannot be imposed by someone else. Also, it needs to be understood that a potential learner's motivation will automatically be directed toward the most pressing need at the moment (Pohl, 1973, p. 16). Even though the CNS cannot *make* a person be motivated, there are some strategies the CNS can use to stimulate motivation. First, identify what the person or group's most pressing concern is at the time. Second, offer incentives whenever possible. Third, include the learners in setting the objectives so that the learning will be useful to them and therefore satisfying. Fourth, organize the material to be learned in a way that is meaningful, such as relating new information to that which is already known. Fifth, make the objectives realistic to the learner. Remember, success is more predictably motivating than failure (Redman, 1984, p. 47). These strategies reflect general principles of motivation. They are all interrelated, and frequently several of them can be utilized at the same time in a single teaching session.

CASE EXAMPLE.   A medical unit of a large hospital began to have increasing numbers of patients admitted with autoimmune deficiency syndrome (AIDS). The nurses were frightened, and some refused to care for these patients. Other nurses then became angry at these co-workers. Amid the dissention, they all agreed that they lacked information and asked the medical CNS to provide an inservice program. The CNS knew what their main concern was (fear of contracting the disease) and planned the inservice to address this issue. The content was organized in a way that related the new information (on AIDS) to the nurses' previous knowledge of communicable disease, infection control, and isolation procedures. The incentive was to learn how not to contract the disease. Since the nurses were emotionally involved (internally motivated) and had requested the inservice (ready to learn), it was a very successful learning experience.

3. *Learning May Occur through Imitation.*

As a mother crab and her child
were strolling along the beach,
the mother crab complained,
"Why, child, do you not walk as
the other creatures — forward
instead of backwards?"

"Why, mother dear," replied the
little crab, "do but set the
example yourself and I will
follow you."

Moral: Example is the best
precept.

AESOP'S FABLES

The CNS is in an excellent position to initiate the learning process through example (role modeling). This is done most frequently in an informal way on a day-to-day basis and is one reason the direct patient care aspect of the CNS role is so important. While giving expert care to patients, other nurses can watch, learn, and hopefully imitate the CNS. Role modeling can also be a planned teaching strategy as in a formal demonstration or an informal example-setting activity. An important concept to remember is that since a CNS is generally considered to be an authority, others will be likely to follow the example that is set regardless of whether it is good or bad. If there is a discrepancy between what is being taught and what the teacher does, the learner will always believe the behavior rather than the words. When the nurse does not exemplify good health habits, the patient's reaction may well be "What you *do* speaks so loudly that I can't hear what you are saying" (Pohl, 1973, p. 12). This adds another responsibility to the CNS as teacher. A cardiovascular CNS may spend several sessions at the community health center with a patient who has severe hypertension explaining risk factors related to his hypertension and the importance of avoiding these risks. If the patient sees the CNS in a fast-food restaurant eating a hamburger and french fries, drinking coffee, and smoking a cigarette, he most likely will decide that it was not all *that* important to avoid those things. The moral is that teaching can be nullified in one moment of observed contradictory behavior of the teacher.

4. *Effective Learning Requires Active Participation.*   The more a person becomes actively involved in the learning process, the more likely it is that the individual will learn. Active involvement, plus utilizing several of the senses, also helps the person retain what was learned longer. Frequently, nurses give out information without taking time to allow the patient to participate, to ask questions, or to practice. This applies to staff learning also. It is not enough to merely *tell* a nurse or intern how to do an unfamiliar procedure. Chances are they will forget parts of what was said by the time they get to the patient's room. For example, when teaching a skill or procedure, allow the new nurse to observe it being done; perhaps provide literature that is relevant; encourage questions; have her assist with the procedure (hands on) and then perform it independently; and give feedback. Active participation is also important when the learning is primarily cognitive rather than psychomotor. Again, encourage questions, comments, and discussion. Get the learners involved! Perhaps have each give a short report related to the topic. Remember, the greater the involvement, the better the learning.

5. *Reinforcement Strengthens Learning.*   Reinforcement is necessary for almost all learning and is of major importance in the learning process. A positive reinforcer is a reward — something that strengthens a specific behavior and increases the probability of its recurrence. A negative reinforcer is any type of "punishment" whose termination will strengthen behavior, that is, the reduction of pain is a negative reinforcer. Negative reinforcement also includes simply the absence of anything positive.

It is well known that nurses generally receive little praise and few pats on the back. Many RNs feel they have had a good day if they have not been criticized, and they learn to keep the IVs on time, give satisfactory care, and make sure the charting is complete in order to avoid criticism. This is negative reinforcement; however, learning does occur. This approach does little to improve the psychological atmosphere of the unit or the spirit of the individual nurse. How much better it would be to encourage learning through positive reinforcement — praise, smiles, pats on the back, perhaps special privileges. The CNS is in a perfect position to do this. The flexibility of the role allows the CNS to move about the unit, make many observations on the quality of care given, and take time to follow up on what was taught, say, in an inservice and time to give recognition of a job well done. To simply say "Helen, you did a nice job with that dressing change" takes no time at all, but it might be the best thing that happened to Helen all day. Also, because the CNS is known to be an expert, praise coming from this source is highly valued. So it is likely that Helen will continue to do a "nice dressing change."

There are so many ways to provide positive reinforcement. All that is needed is the decision to do it, a little creativity, and follow-through. One surgical CNS in a large county hospital noticed that many of the nurses did not know how to do a wet-to-dry dressing correctly. She gave an inservice program including a demonstration on the topic and explained the importance of improving their efforts. Later, whenever she observed that a nurse had improved her technique, the CNS presented the nurse with a certificate of recognition for superior achievement and excellence of performance. This had a very positive response. It was always a surprise and was very much appreciated by the staff nurses.

This learning principle of positive reinforcement is very closely linked with the principle of motivation discussed earlier. Hospital and nursing administrators are increasingly recognizing the value of increased learning for their nurses. Today, nurses are receiving incentives or rewards (positive reinforcement) for education—extra pay for certification and master's degrees, time off with pay to attend workshops, and opportunity to advance up a clinical ladder, which means added prestige and, again, increased salary.

This same principle is important in patient education also. Positive reinforcement repeated over time could help improve patient adherence to treatment. The patient cannot receive money for learning correct health behavior, but the payoff can be receiving praise, feeling more in control, or gaining improved health. Each new concept or skill learned by the patient should be reinforced by praise, special privilege, a certificate, or some other means. For the child, there are many possibilities for reward—games, balloons, stickers, comic books, and so on. A diabetic person who has correctly learned his meal plan and exchanges could be permitted to go to the cafeteria to select his own foods.

These learning principles are rules that universally apply to all teaching situations and will be extremely helpful in planning learning activities.

PRACTICAL CONSIDERATIONS

Attributes Necessary for the CNS Teacher

Teaching in the role of a CNS is different from teaching students in the classroom. Nurses are sometimes resistant to change and prefer to keep doing things "as we've always done them." They "don't have time" to listen or attend inservice programs. Patients are too sick and are discharged before there is a chance to teach them. They try to be "good patients" and say, "Yes I understand" when they do not understand. Some would rather watch the soap operas on television than attend diabetes classes. So, in addition to the usual characteristics needed for classroom teaching (see Figure 6.2), the CNS also needs the following special attributes:

1. *Patience.* Changing attitudes, habits, and perhaps life-styles takes time. Others may not place the same importance on new information as you do. You may say the same thing several times with no change occurring. It is necessary to continue to be supportive through several attempts. It might also be necessary to help the nurse or the patient to *want* to change, and sometimes this takes a long time. But if the results are important, they are worth waiting for.

2. *Perseverance.* This is similar to patience but a more active patience. A person can be patient by sitting and waiting, but to move ahead with an educational program, the CNS may have to actively persevere in overcoming roadblocks. It might mean persistent follow-through of each step, phone calls, or if other educators are involved, such as dieticians, meetings and organizing. Perseverance means never giving up.

3. *Nonjudgmental.* Being nonjudgmental means accepting people for where they are now and not making their shortcomings into a sin or something of which one disapproves. In her lighthearted treatise on diabetes education, Tupling (1981) reminds us, "It's not a sin to be fat . . . It's not silly to be frightened of needles. It's not bad or stupid to ignore the diet. It's not crazy or irresponsible to forget an insulin injection," (p. 81).

Students Perceptions	Administrator's Perceptions
1. Organization/clarity	1. Being well prepared for class
2. Enthusiasm/stimulation	2. Motivating students to do their best
3. Instructor knowledge	3. Communicating effectively to the level of the student
4. Clinical competence	4. Demonstrating comprehensive knowledge
5. Clinical supervision	5. Treating students with respect
6. Group instructional skill	

Figure 6.2. Characteristics of effective teaching. (*Compiled from Van Ort, S., Journal of Nursing Education, Vol. 22, No. 8, October 1983, pp. 324–328.*)

Frequently, judgments are ways of generalizing about people in a way that

1. is not necessarily based on adequate information,
2. is not likely to result in being an effective "helper" for the client, and
3. allows the person to be labeled and discarded as being a resistive or hopeless client (Tupling, 1981, p. 82).

4. *Creativity.*   Imagination and creativity are invaluable assets for the CNS teacher, both for planning teaching strategies and for inventing interesting incentives for learning. Imagination is often required when a special need arises, such as when a patient is blind, or illiterate, or does not speak English. All barriers can be overcome or circumvented with enough creativity.

The ability to be creative serves another purpose also. When the CNS is responsible for teaching the same topic over and over, such as in orientation sessions, nurse internship programs, or diabetes education, there is a high risk of boredom for the CNS. When this happens, the teaching will also be boring, so it is time to step back and take a fresh look at what is being taught. Are there more interesting strategies that could be used? Is there a new approach that might be more stimulating? Creativity can serve the dual purpose of helping to assure that the teaching–learning process will be interesting for both the learner and the teacher.

5. *Flexibility.*   Rarely does any teaching session happen exactly as planned in a busy hospital setting. The CNS needs to be able to adapt quickly to the changing needs and situations that arise for staff and patients. If the CNS is rigid in the what, when, and where of what is taught, it indicates that her goals are more important than the learners' goals. Both will end up being disappointed and frustrated. An example of a flexible CNS follows. A pediatric clinical nurse specialist had planned an inservice on infant feeding. As the nurses arrived, they were talking excitedly and with much concern about a little 3 year old that had just been admitted with several injuries. They suspected abuse but were not sure how to assess it or document it or what their legal responsibility was. Being sensitive to the mood and concerns of the nurses and remembering that the best moment for learning to occur is when a problem is recognized by the learner, she closed her folder of notes on infant feeding and gave an impromptu inservice program on child abuse.

6. *Sense of Humor.*   At times it is possible to get caught up in taking oneself too seriously. Effective education *is* serious, but it is also lively, entertaining, and fun. When teaching is no longer fun, something is wrong, and if the teacher no longer enjoys the sessions, probably no one else will either. Having a sense of humor does not mean being a clown or laughing or joking all the time. It simply means taking things as they come and accepting them for what they are without becoming defensive, frustrated or angry.

7. *Enthusiasm.*   Picture the cheerleaders at a high school football game — jumping, yelling, clapping, cheering. The amount of energy and vitality generated comes from enthusiasm in what they believe — their school winning. At times the CNS teacher needs to be a cheerleader — to encourage, to reinforce, and to inspire learning. Enthusiasm for teaching is the necessary ingredient that stimulates the previously mentioned attributes of creativity, flexibility, and humor. It is the fuel that maintains the teacher's motivation and ability to sustain interest in the teaching–learning process.

TEACHING GUIDELINES

While there are many, many books written on how to teach and many variations of strategies depending on what is being taught, there are a number of guidelines described by Toth (1983, p. 32) that seem appropriate in all teaching situations. These guidelines include the following concepts that facilitate the teaching–learning process:

1. *Known to Unknown.*   This emphasizes the importance of assessment. What does the patient already know about his disease or condition? What is the staff nurse's previous experience or knowledge base about the topic. Begin there and move on to the new information (Toth, 1983, p. 32).

2. *Simple to Complex.*   It is helpful to start with ideas that are easy to understand and build on them and expand them to more difficult concepts. A person with diabetes may not be able to understand the complex mechanism of carbohydrate metabolism and insulin requirement but can start by learning that when food is eaten, it turns to sugar and enters the bloodstream. The instruction can increase in complexity from there.

3. *Self-pacing.*   Each person learns at a different rate so the timing of instruction should be individualized as much as possible. This is easier to

accomplish in a one-to-one teaching situation and may be difficult in groups, but it always needs to be considered and planned for.

4. *Whole before Parts.* An example of this method is especially clear when teaching procedures or skills. When teaching a patient colostomy care, for example, it is best to demonstrate the *entire* procedure first. This gives the patient an overview of what the end results are to be. Then each component can be taught step by step until the whole procedure is learned. The sequence then is: whole—parts—whole.

5. *Space Out Practice.* The attention span of most learners is said to be about 20 minutes. When a person is uncomfortable, anxious, or overly distracted, as in a hospital, the attention time is shorter. If a patient needs to learn a procedure or treatment before being discharged, it is important to identify this early in the hospital stay so that there is time to space out the practice of the skill. The CNS who *knows the trajectory* will anticipate this and begin the following:

- Teaching gradually.
- Having patient exercise muscle groups so he or she can get out of bed, balance, and use crutches.

Spacing allows for repetition and will enhance retention.

6. *Transfer Learning.* Positive transfer usually occurs when two learning tasks contain enough similarities that one task facilitates the learning of another. For example, if a student nurse has learned to give a subcutaneous injection, she will most likely be able to give an intramuscular injection. If common characteristics can be pointed out, it can ease learning (Kleffner, 1980).

7. *Varied Methods.* The teaching method depends on the content, the learners, materials, available space, and so on. The usual teaching methods are listed in Table 6.1, but the variety is limited only by the amount of creativity in the teacher.

There are two main areas of teaching in which the CNS will be involved: staff/student education and patient/family education. The teaching–learning theories, principles, and guidelines previously mentioned apply to both groups, but there are special considerations that need to be emphasized regarding each.

TABLE 6.1. Teaching Approaches

Approach	Advantages	Disadvantages
Written teaching aids	Permanent record the learner can refer to Efficient, assures that important points are covered Complex thoughts can be expressed better in writing	Readability of written materials is frequently too high for intended audience Often overused by health professionals, overreliance may decrease learning Written materials at best supplement other methods; usually not effective when used alone.
Group instruction	Economical and efficient, can teach a number of individuals at one time Provides peer support reinforcement and social pressure Increases opportunities for self-rewards Decreases feelings of isolation	Some people may have problems that cannot be dealt with adequately in a group Some may resent loss of privacy in group Nurse may not be as comfortable or effective leading groups
Lecture (giving advice or instructions)	Useful when objective is to get accurate, factual information to learner Efficient, simple, straightforward Good in situations where rapid instructions are necessary	Communication often impersonal (nurse dominated) Method may not allow for questions Often not able to assure that learner understands Method often overused by health professionals At best people may only remember half of what they are told
Discussion, one-to-one counseling	Increases learner involvement Able to make adaptations and compromises based on learner's perceptions Can individualize, often more learner oriented	If objectives or goals are not clear, conversations may lack direction, vital information may be missed, and desired learning may not occur

113

TABLE 6.1. *Continued*

Approach	Advantages	Disadvantages
Roleplaying (rehearsal of desired behaviors)	Provides for transfer of learning; learner can "try out" new behaviors, skills, or attitudes Provides opportunity for nurse to evaluate learning When nurse or others in a group roleplays, patients are encouraged to model new behaviors Increases learner involvement	May be more time consuming Requires more skill than advice giving or one-to-one counseling Nurse or patient may not feel comfortable with the technique
Demonstration (practice and redemonstration)	Good for learning motor skills Assists nurse-teacher in evaluating learning	May take more time than other methods Hospitalized patient may be too sick, too tired, or too involved with other tests or treatments to adequately practice a needed skill
Audiovisual teaching aids (films, slides, cassette tapes, overhead transparencies, or records	Can be used over and over (increases retention) Provides standard content Efficient, may take place of repetitious information giving May be able to simulate actual situations better than a live demonstration due to constraints of teaching environment Can visualize various angles, close-ups, etc., that actual demonstrations may not be able to Brief videotapes can often be successfully used to "trigger" discussions Patients can often identify with characters in AV programs; provides for modeling, transfer of learning	Can be overused and impersonal if used alone Better as a supplement to other methods May be expensive Staff may not know how to use equipment May not have a place to use or store equipment

Compiled from Toth, S., *Patient Teaching: A Nursing Process Approach*, Westport CT, J.B. Lippincott, 1983, pp. 33–34.

Staff Education

Teaching other health professionals, either formally in groups or informally on a one-to-one, impromptu basis, has its frustrations and its rewards. To keep the scale tipped in favor of the rewards, it might be helpful to keep a few points in mind.

1. Make every effort to establish or maintain a good relationship with the staff nurses. Thay are professionals and will resent being talked down to. Treat them as colleagues in a respectful, sharing way rather than in a preaching way.

2. Be sure you know what you are talking about. You will be spotted in a minute if you try faking it. Prepare adequately for the presentation if it's a formal one, but again, do not lecture. Your knowledge base should be sufficient to be able to encourage and respond to questions without having everything written down.

3. Recognize the knowledge of others. If you have been asked to present a topic that is not exactly in your field of expertise, ask the group if any of them have special experience or knowledge of the topic and invite them to participate by answering questions for you or adding comments. You could switch your role to one of discussion leader rather than teacher. You do not *always* have to be the expert!

4. Encourage staff nurses to share their expertise with their peers, and give them responsibility to assist in providing staff education, perhaps on a rotating basis. This should be done in a way that is not interpreted as just an addition to the work load but as a recognition that they are knowledgeable professionals. It can be something as simple as asking the nurse to share a case example of a specific "difficult" patient with the group and discuss the problems and solutions that occurred.

5. There will be times when you have worked very hard to plan and present an inservice program and no one shows up. This is a pitfall that happens at *least* once to every CNS. Maintain a sense of humor. Do not get angry, depressed, or defensive; instead, try to identify what kept people away. Perhaps the topic was not pertinent to their needs. Maybe the topic was *very* pertinent, but they are expressing resistance to change by staying away. It might merely be that the timing was off. The most common reason nurses give for not attending an inservice is "not enough time" or "so busy I forgot."

Whatever the reason, do not take it personally, but do try to assess the reason and change it. "Not having enough time" brings us to the next point.

6. Nurses are very busy people, and they do have difficulty getting away from their patients, so the more creative the CNS can be in providing ways to disseminate information at the convenience of all the more this will enhance the inservice and continuing education concept. For example, the nurses lounge on each unit is an excellent place to communicate with the staff.

One CNS designed eye-catching posters (a new one each month) with both new and review information on various topics and posted it in the nurses' lounge. One poster was a review of hyperalimentation. It had a series of questions with corresponding flaps that when lifted revealed the answers. A bulletin board titled "What's New In Patient Care" could be installed so that current articles or items of interest could be posted. Another CNS placed a loose leaf binder on the table in the lounge. It was titled "The Weekly Reader," and each week she placed one or two new pertinent articles in it. The nurses were able to leisurely read the articles during coffee break or lunch. Providing short, audio-cassette tapes is another way for nurses to get information at their own convenience. They can listen to the tapes at the hospital or check them out and take them home. They can even listen to them in the car on the way home.

These are just a few of the many ways that staff education can be made available in a time-efficient way. Yet, at times, it seems that no matter what you do, the staff will not participate. In Bivin's (1973) discussion of why staff education programs are poorly attended, she points out that it is invariably because traditional programs do not meet the needs of the adult learner. An adult will not learn until he feels the need for a particular knowledge or skill. Therefore, it is important to find out where the staff wants to go in terms of their own development. Once they choose a goal of their own, it becomes their responsibility, as much as the clinical specialist's, to meet the goal. They will begin to become actively involved. It is at this point, says Bivin (1973, p. 719), that the CNS will be of great assistance:

> She often will be able to simplify their learning and make the attainment of the goals less haphazard and more quickly realized than would be possible without her. Surely this is the essence of teaching — and may well be one of the most valuable roles a clinical specialist can adopt.

The key issue then is to keep in mind the characteristics of the adult learner, as described by Knowles (1980), and all the implications associated with these characteristics (see Table 6.2). These guidelines will provide a very useful framework for developing successful staff education programs.

Student Education

Clincial nurse specialists are frequently involved in student education, either informally because students just happen to be there or formally as a preceptor for graduate students or as instructor for undergraduate students. In a joint appointment, the CNS has a very specific responsibility for teaching an assigned number of students specified content and for evaluating their performance and assigning a grade. While this involves a much more formal student–teacher relationship than does staff or patient evaluation, all of the previously discussed principles and guidelines still apply. Professional students are adults, so keeping the characteristics of adult learners in mind will facilitate their learning.

Because of her clinical expertise, the CNS has the opportunity to clearly influence the level of performance and knowledge of not only nursing students but also medical students and to encourage nursing and medical students to collaborate in planning quality patient care. When a student nurse can observe the CNS in a collegial relationship with physicians, it will foster improved nurse–physician relationships in the future, breaking down the old barriers that have historically hindered communication.

In some health science centers it is not uncommon for medical and nursing students to be enrolled in the same courses, especially electives. These

TABLE 6.2.   Characteristics of Adult Learners

---

1.   The adult must want to learn and feel the need for a particular knowledge or skill.
2.   Adults like learning based on active involvement.
3.   Adult learning is facilitated by an environment in which there is freedom to question and disagree.
4.   Adults desire guidance and feedback on progress.
5.   Adult learning is facilitated by an informal environment.

Compiled from Neissner, P., *Nursing Leadership*, Vol. 2, No. 1, 1979, p. 21–30.

courses are jointly taught by medical and nursing faculty and usually cover such topics as ethical issues, psychosocial aspects, communication skills, and basic procedures (venipuncture, sterile technique, etc.). The CNS is in a perfect position to be formally involved in teaching medical students along with nursing students in these multidisciplinary courses. In the clinical component of these courses, CNSs have joined with their physician colleagues in co-teaching during clinical conferences, patient care rounds, and even home visits.

When it comes to teaching students, however, *nursing* students will always be the CNS's first priority. There are special rewards for the CNS in seeing a new nursing student grow and learn, accept responsibility, and blossom into a "full-fledged nurse." It is one of those inner rewards that make classroom teaching and clinical instruction of students very satisfying.

Patient and Family Education

Patient education has long been recognized as an essential component of quality, comprehensive patient care, and the Nurse Practice Acts of most states reflect health care teaching as a function of the nurse. In recent years, more and more emphasis is being placed on the importance of patient education as not only the responsibility of health care providers but the right of the patient. Accrediting agencies such as the Joint Commission for Accreditation of Hospitals (JCAH, 1983) have established standards that require evidence that patient and family teaching is being done. The American Hospital Association (AHA) has drafted a patient's bill of rights, which states the patient has the right to obtain "complete current information concerning his diagnosis, treatment and prognosis in terms the patient can be reasonably expected to understand" (Billie, 1981, p. 5). Health care consumers have become much more sophisticated in their knowledge of health and disease, and when an individual is hospitalized, he wants and expects to learn about his condition. Today, with the trend being to shorten the length of hospital stay due to the DRG approach to reimbursement, patients are going home sooner, so it is extremely important for the patient and his family to have enough information to be able to safely manage his care at home.

Although there is no question that patient teaching is necessary, there still seems to be a serious problem in providing adequate education for patients.

While there are many excellent, structured programs being offered in hospitals for certain groups, such as diabetics and cardiac patients, the day-to-day instruction for most patients is left to chance. Why is this so? The most common reason given by nurses is, of course, lack of time. Another reason is that they are not sure *what* to teach (uncomfortable with the content), and others feel they do not know *how* to teach (uncomfortable in the role). Probably one of the most common unspoken reasons is that many nurses have the feeling, "What's the use?" Far too often nurses have been frustrated when, after spending much time and effort teaching a patient, they find the patient is admitted again at a later date not remembering anything of what had been taught. This frustrating occurrence is an example of the difficulty of learning under stress and the fact that teaching does not ensure learning.

Much of what has been said about staff education applies to adult patient education as well, especially the importance of utilizing the characteristics of adult learners. Nurses tend to relate to patients in a parenting way, talking to them as children, and while it is true that during hospitalization some regression may occur in terms of dependency and helplessness, the adult patient remains an adult, and teaching efforts need to reflect the principles of adult learning.

The CNS can help to solve some of the problems related to patient teaching in several ways. First, the CNS can assume the responsibility for all patient teaching. Needless to say, this is unrealistic because the CNS cannot be available at all times, and teaching needs to occur at the time questions are asked, 24 hours a day, 7 days per week. If one person (the CNS) is identified as the "patient educator," the other nurses will be less interested and will assume that patient teaching is no longer their responsibility. A second approach described by Malkin and Louteri (1980) is the "decentralized approach." Here *all* nursing and health personnel are utilized for education. The advantages are that everyone assumes responsibility, and a maximum number of patients and families can be educated. The disadvantage is that, as noted earlier, some nurses do not have the skill or confidence to teach. The solution to this revolves around the CNS's role as educator. The CNS can help them learn how, what, and when to teach and how to involve the learner and assess learning needs. Developing instructional outlines, selecting audiovisual aids, and organizing materials are examples of CNS assistance. But the CNS should not relegate all actual teaching to the staff. The role of the CNS as role model is very important, and the example of bedside teaching is valuable (Bivins, 1973).

One of the major differences between patient education and staff/student education is that the patient is sick, possibly frightened, and in a strange environment. All of these are barriers to learning and are reasons for the patient not to remember what is taught. Therefore, in addition to the general guidelines previously discussed, there are several practical points to keep in mind.

1. Always begin with a thorough assessment. What does the patient *need* to know (the survival skills)? What does he already know? What does he *want* to know? What is he capable of learning based on his present physical and psychological condition? Nothing succeeds like success—so start with tasks patients can be successful at! What are patient goals, what does he want to do: Be able to (a) walk to the store to get a newspaper and (b) travel to see his daughter and grandchildren. To achieve (a), he needs to do 1, 2, 3. To achieve (b), he needs to do 5, 6, 7. If the patient understands how activities *relate* to his goal—that is a motivator! Assessment is essential.

2. Always include family members when possible. The family is often very anxious to know what is going on and to help. They will be valuable reinforcers and supporters for the patient and in some cases will be responsible for taking over the care when the patient is discharged.

3. Use the patient's own language and avoid medical terminology. Even if the patient can speak English, if his first language is, say, Spanish, it might be necessary to teach in Spanish. Under stress, many people comprehend better in their native language. Also remember that many words that are common to health professionals may not be understood by patients (see Table 6.3).

4. Always develop a written plan based on the assessment of the patient's learning needs. This can be a preprinted form or checklist or individually written as part of the nursing care plan. This written plan provides for continuity from one shift to the next and provides written documentation.

5. Use multiple short teaching sessions rather than a few longer ones. The ill person's attention span is short, so 5 minutes may be more effective than 30. A session of 5–10 minutes is also more reasonable for the busy nurse. For example, each time the patient is given medication, he can be given some instruction, that is, name, dose, side effects. The next time he can be asked to repeat what he learned. By the time of discharge, the patient will then know what he needs to know about the medication.

TABLE 6.3. Common Medical Terminology

Commonly Misunderstood Words	Alternate Wording
Ambulate	Walk
Void	Pass urine, pass water
Respiratory	Breathing, lungs
Uterus	Womb, place where baby grows
Postpartum	After the baby comes
Genitals	Bottom, private parts
Carbohydrate	Starchy foods
Cathartic	Medicine to loosen bowels
Orally	Taken in mouth
Persists	Keeps up, lasts
Diagnosis	Problem
Inject	Put inside with needle
Instill	Put inside
Complications	Later problems, further problems
Contraindicated	Not allowed, to be avoided

6. Quiz the patient or in some way evaluate that the learning objectives are being met. Frequent verbal quizzing is very effective if done in a nonthreatening way. And if the patient is forewarned that he will be quizzed, it tends to increase his attentiveness. For example, after telling a diabetic patient that normal blood glucose is 70–120 mg/dl. the nurse might say, "I want you to try to remember that normal blood sugar is 70–120. This afternoon I'll come back to see you and I'll ask you to tell me." Then be true to your word and go back and ask. If you fail to follow up on a quiz, the patient will not be as attentive next time.

7. Always give positive feedback for each new learning task accomplished.

8. Be sure to identify a patient's special needs. Every patient is different, and every age group needs a different approach. Do not indiscriminately pass out pamphlets. The patient may not be able to read because of language or visual problems or because of a low literacy level. Doak and Doak (1985), in their excellent book *Teaching Patients With Low Literacy Skills*, point out that 20% of the adult American population have reading skills below the fifth-grade level and are considered functionally illiterate. This special need may require innovative teaching strategies.

9. Make effective use of "self" to establish rapport and positive interactions in order to have a partnership with the patient and family in planning and providing health education.

The teaching role can be the most rewarding of all the CNS roles and at the same time the most frustrating. The rewarding part is when you have given an inservice program that has stimulated the nurses to make a change that will improve patient care or when a patient tells you how much better he feels now that you have explained his treatments. The frustrating part is when, 3 months after the inservice program, the staff begins to revert back to old habits or the patient continues to sneak candy after you meticulously explained his diet. Fortunately, the rewards far outnumber the frustrations, and seeing an improvement in the patient's care or health status makes it all worthwhile.

BIBLIOGRAPHY

Banta, J. (1979). Definition of community health. *Community health today and tomorrow* (p. 12). New York: National League of Nursing.

Bigge, M.L. (1971). *Learning theories for teachers*. New York: Harper & Row.

Billie, D. A. (1981). *Practical approach to patient teaching*. Boston: Little, Brown.

Bivins, V. (1973, December). The clinical specialist—an educator. *Nursing Clinics of North America*, **8**(4), 715–721.

Boylan, A. (1983, October 12). Specialist teaching. *Nursing Times*, **79**, 45–46.

Christman, L. (1979, March/April). The practitioner teacher. *Nurse Educator*, 8–11.

Doak, C., & Doak, L. (1985). *Teaching patients with low literacy skills*. Philadelphia: Lippincott.

Draye, M. A., & Pesznecker, B. (1980, September/October). Teaching activities of family nurse practitioners. *Nurse Practitioner*, **5**(28), 28.

Falvo, D. (1985). *Effective patient education: A guide to increased compliance*. Rockville, MD: Aspen Systems.

Floyd, G. J. (1982). Qualities/characteristics preferred in continuing education instructors. *Journal of Continuing Education in Nursing*, **13**(3), 5–14.

JCAH Manual (1983). Chicago: Joint Commission on Accreditation of Hospitals.

Kleffner, J. (1980). *The teaching learning process* (p. 104). San Antonio, TX: The University of Texas Health Science Center at San Antonio.

Knowles, M. S. (1984). *The adult learner: A neglected species* (3rd ed.). Houston: Gulf.

Knowles, M. S. (1980). *The modern practice of adult education: From pedagogy to androgogy* (2nd ed.). New York: Cambridge.

Little, B. (1982, August 4). Sharing good ideas. *Nursing Mirror*, **5**(155), ii–iv.

Malkin, S., & Lauteri, P. (1980). A community hospital's approach: Decentralized patient education. *Nursing Administration Quarterly*, **2**(4), 101–105.

Pohl, M. L. (1973). *The teaching function of the nursing practitioner*. Duburque, IA: Brown.

Rankin, S. H., & Duffy, K. (1983). *Patient education: Issues, principles, and guidelines*. Philadelphia: Lippincott.

Redman, E. (1984). *The process of patient teaching in nursing* (p. 47). St. Louis: Mosby.

Rufo, K. L. (1981). Guidelines for inservice education for registered nurses. *Journal of Continuing Education*, **12**(1), 26–33.

Toth, S. (1983). *Patient teaching: A nursing process approach*. Philadelphia: Lippincott.

Tupling, H. (1981). *You've got to get through the outside layer: A handbook for health educators using diabetes as a model*. Published by Diabetes Education and Assessment Programme of the Royal North Shore Hospital of Sydney and The Northern Metropolitan Health Region of the Health Commission of New South Wales. Printed and distributed in the United States by the American Association of Diabetes Educators and Ames Division of Miles Laboratories.

Van Ort, S. (1983, October). Developing a system for documenting teaching effectiveness. *Journal of Nursing Education*, **22**(8), 324–328.

Wise, P. S. Y. (1980). Adult teaching strategies. *Journal of Continuing Education in Nursing*, **11**(6), 15–17.

CASE STUDY: THE CNS AS TEACHER
Diana Huston-Anderson, M.S.N., R.N.

I entered into a position as a CNS directly from an academic background. My 5 years of faculty work and numerous years as a teaching assistant in schools of nursing were appropriate and a most necessary preparation for the role of a CNS at St. Paul Medical Center in Dallas, Texas.

A primary goal has been to develop a comprehensive arthritis center at St. Paul. This means a program that encompasses outpatient education, community education, inpatient education, staff education, and eventually research. The center concept at St. Paul is defined as a facility that serves as a "hub" for all arthritis patients at the various stages of illness, (i.e., newly diagnosed, postoperative, rehabilitative states). The thrust of the center is aimed at providing health care education with an emphasis on preventative health and promotion of the individuals responsibility for self-management.

The CNS serves as coordinator of a multidisciplinary team and is responsible for conducting a needs assessment of the arthritis population, curriculum development, program implementation and evaluation, as well as initiation and follow-through of many marketing strategies. As can be seen, this position places heavy emphasis on the specialist's knowledge of the educational process.

Discussion will focus on those aspects of the position that directly require skills as "teacher." One of those aspects is the coordination of the teaching efforts of the multidisciplinary team. Initially, this required a great deal of time with respect to program development and program delivery. Though extremely knowledgeable in their specific areas, this group of health professionals often lacked understanding of development of goals, objectives, and content in their respective fields. When asked to formally present content to patients in the classroom setting, some also lacked experience with delivery of information. It was necessary for the CNS to serve as the "expert" in those areas and to guide the team, in a sense teaching the team to teach!

After evaluating the teams' effectiveness of presentation, I became aware that not all of the health professionals were interested in or equipped to instruct in a classroom situation. Based on the participants, the staff, and evaluation of classes, it was at times necessary to allow a team member to "trade off" their teaching responsibilities with another member of the group. In this situation, that team member usually was able to contribute in another role within the auspices of the team.

To further illustrate the team approach, it might be helpful to describe the group. The arthritis team is comprised of a medical director and assistant medical director, both M.D.'s and rheumatologists, two physical therapists, an occupational therapist, social worker, pharmacist, registered dietitian, orthopedic nurse, a lay chairman of our support group, secretary, administrator, and the CNS.

Obviously, with such a large group, the effective coordination of the team becomes paramount. In this setting, the CNS certainly cannot function optimally without an effective team. A monthly team meeting is directed by the CNS to assess progress, discuss patients, and look at problem areas. I also meet one to one on a regular basis both formally and informally with team members to discuss specific details of program development, evaluate progress, and so on.

The time the arthritis team allocates to the arthritis center is contracted through the various department heads. The coordinator of the team must keep in mind the demands on the team within the medical center and within their own departments. At times this can be frustrating as team members cannot leave their responsibilities to attend team meetings or meet deadlines as planned. Also, the evaluation process must be handled carefully because team members are not directly responsible to the CNS.

Obviously, assembling the team and developing quality programs must be completed before patients are sought or introduced to the center. The best way to define the progress of the arthritis center may be to outline the programs that are in place and show how they have branched from one another within the last year (Figure 6.3). The stages of development in such a variety of programs has indeed been a challenge.

A second and major aspect of the role is the actual direct patient teaching in which I am involved. Again, this has been challenging and at times has required *all* my skill and experience in teaching. I have found myself teaching swimming programs and exercise routines, acting in videotapes and writing scripts, pinch hitting for absent team members with only minutes notice, instructing and making assessments over the telephone, and at times putting in 4–5 hours of actual lecture time in one day!

The Arthritis Aquatic Program
6 weeks, 3 times per week, low fees

The Arthritis Self-help Course
6-week program, 2 hours per week

Both cosponsored by the Arthritis Foundation

Out-patient Programs Developed at St. Paul	The St. Paul Arthritis Support Group	In-Patient Programs for St. Paul
THE ARTHRITIS CENTER PATIENT EDUCATION SERIES	Meet once a month. Free program coordinated by clinical nurse specialist and a patient committee.	Consultation by clinical nurse specialist upon physician referral.
A 9-week program, 2 hours per week, taught by the Arthritis Team.	Consultations	Beginning video taping of Patient Education Series to show in patient rooms.
The Arthritis Weight Loss and Exercise Program	Physical therapy Occupational therapy Nutrition Relaxation/pain management Social work	Physician's referral to attend Patient Education Series while hospitalized.
8 weeks of class 2 hours per week 8 weeks of maintenance includes physical therapy, dietitian	Staff Education	
	Word of mouth by team. Structured inservices by clinical nurse specialist. Clinical nurse specialist as resource and consultant to staff.	

Figure 6.3. Community service programs.

Other tasks I have undertaken directly related to patient teaching include building a collection of books for a patient library, designing media creatively for use in class, and forming a "media library." Another area of responsibility has been to select what audiovisual equipment is necessary as well as what materials are appropriate for patient and staff use.

This position at St. Paul has been a unique opportunity to develop a concept from the "ground up." Administration has given me free reign to develop programs and use creative teaching methods. I have grown personally and truly feel I am functioning in an expanded role. Of course, there have been conflicts along the way but none so steep that they outweigh the autonomy and satisfaction provided by the CNS role.

7

THE CNS AS CONSULTANT

Shirley W. Menard, M.S.N., R.N.

Chapter Objectives

At the conclusion of this chapter, the reader will:

1. State the purpose and types of consultation.
2. Understand the role of the consultant in the consultative process.
3. Discuss the ways in which the CNS can implement the role of consultant.

THEORETICAL PERSPECTIVES

Caplan (1970 p. 19) has described consultation as:

> a process of interaction between two professional persons — the consultant, who
> is a specialist, and the consultee, who invokes the consultant's help in regard
> to a current work problem with which she's having some difficulty and which
> she has decided is within the other's area of specialized competence.

Consultation is quite different from collaboration, which may allow active participation by the CNS. In consultation, there is no active participation by the consultant, and the consultee is free to accept or reject any or all of the consultant's recommendations.

Caplan (1970) identifies four basic types of consultation. Client-centered case consultation involves the management of a specific patient. For instance, the CNS may be asked by several staff nurses how to care for a patient following open heart surgery. Consultee-centered case consultation involves the use of the consultant by the consultee to help the consultee with a difficult area of case management. For example, a staff nurse consults with the CNS on how the staff nurse can best teach the mother of a baby with cleft palate how to feed that baby. Program-centered administrative consultation involves the planning and development of new programs or the improvement of existing programs. For example, the CNS may be asked by the head nurse to consult on the development of an orientation program for new staff. Consultation in the consultee-centered administrative consultation deals with the problems the consultee may have in developing and organizing programs. For example, the Director of Inservice may consult with the CNS on a specific area of an educational program she is developing in which the CNS is seen as an expert. The CNS may find herself involved in any or all of these types of consultation depending on her area of expertise.

Boehm (1956) has identified six elements that are parts of the consultation:

1. Consultation is a process.
2. The process is educational.
3. The consultant possesses a unique competence that makes her, in relation to the consultee, an expert.
4. Consultation focuses on a problem perceived by the consultee.
5. It is the consultee who initiates the consultation and formulates the problem.
6. Consultation has a "take it or leave it" quality.

These elements would tend to show that the CNS is in a position to be a consultant to other nurses, other members of the health care team, and to patients and/or clients. The CNS is well versed in process and should be able to easily adapt the knowledge to the consultative process. As a teacher, the CNS is aware of teaching and learning principles. Certainly, the CNS is an "expert" in her area of practice with specific skills in that area. Because the problem must be perceived, initiated, and formulated by the consultee, the CNS should be available and approachable. The CNS who is never available to the staff or who places barriers between herself and staff will not be consulted very often. Although a consultee must feel that his perception of the problem is acceptable, there will be occasions when the consultee cannot verbalize the problem. At times the client may verbalize a problem, but some other problem is really the issue. Norris (1977, p. 760) states that "it is probably useful to accept people's diagnosis of their problems without critical . . . questions." The CNS should be able to assist the client to identify the "real" problem(s). Finally, the staff must trust that whatever they decide will be accepted by the consultant even if they decide against the consultant's recommendations.

Sedgwick (1973) has enumerated three kinds of consultants. The *expert* consultant "has unique skills and expertise" (p. 773) that she brings to bear on specific situations. The *resource* consultant "provides relevant information to enable the consultee to make decisions based on the widest range of alternatives." (p. 773) The *process* consultant "brings about changes in the situation that enables the consultee to make decisions." (p. 773) It would appear that the CNS functioning as a process consultant would also be functioning as a change agent. The CNS may be utilized in all of these consultant roles during any one consultation.

Consultation needs to be approached in an orderly manner (see Figure 7.1). The initial request for consultation must come from the consultee. Once the consultation is initiated, the consultant must set about collecting data from all sources. The skilled consultant will pull from her broad theoretical and experiential base to form a working diagnosis of the correct problem(s). The planned action phase has the consultant presenting her recommendations to the consultee. These recommendations may necessitate the putting on of one or more roles by the CNS. Blake (1977) lists the roles of advocate, expert, stimulator, and change agent. The *advocate* believes her recommendations to be absolutely correct and tries to convince the consultee of this. One must be careful in the advocate role not to violate the rule of consultation dealing with the right of the consultee to accept or reject recommendations. The *expert* presents a variety of solutions with supportive theory base. The *stimulator* encourages the consultee to question and probe. The *change agent* "deliberately, systematically collaborates with the consultee to revise an existing practice, procedure or policy to the desired one" (Blake, 1977). After presenting recommendations, the consultant must document her part in the process. This documentation could be via the nurse's notes, patient progress notes, or an official consultation form. The consultee is free to accept or reject any or all of the consultant's recommendations. Evaluation by both the consultant and the consultee is a vital part of the process and may lead to

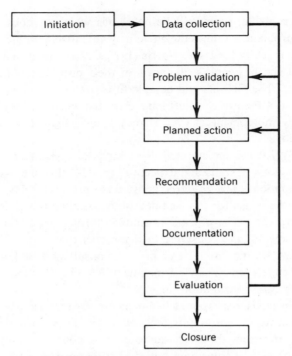

Figure 7.1. Consultation process.

further consultation or to closure. With every consultation, there must be a closure point that is mutually agreeable. This closure point is generally decided upon during the initial phase of the consultation. It must be remembered that closure does not divorce the consultant from the process. The consultant follows up via phone or personally with the consultee to see how things are progressing. This gives the consultee an opening to request further consultation if needed. Utilizing the preceding steps of the consultative process can give the CNS an organized basis for carrying out consultation.

PRACTICAL IMPLICATIONS

The theory of consultation is no help if one is unable to put that theory into action. Consultation is at times difficult for the CNS because it must be initiated by another person. Generally, nurse members of the health care team have not utilized consultation with others, and so the CNS must first help those nurses identify when to consult and how to go about the process of consulting. There are several things that the CNS can do to educate and/ or stimulate other nurses into the consultative process. A brief inservice on consultation is a good starting point. If this is then followed by frequent examples of nursing consultation, it may be easier for staff nurses to begin to assimilate consultation into their routine. Several methods involving consultation may be used to encourage the staff's participation. Weekly nursing rounds may be scheduled at change of shift to discuss specific patient cases and management. This gives the staff nurses the opportunity to begin to identify and verbalize questions, a necessary first step in the consultative process. The second method is the active use of other nurse experts so that staff can see consultation in progress. Still another example is for the CNS to actively consult with and be consulted by other health care professionals. This can frequently be accomplished by making oneself available for rounds with the interdisciplinary team. If the hospital setting where the CNS is employed does not utilize an interdisciplinary approach to patient care, the CNS is in a position to use consultation to implement such an approach. Many novice consultants are not sure exactly what it is they should be doing. There are no easy answers to this problem; however, it is helpful to know generally what the consultant is responsible for and then adapt those generalities to the specific situation. Blumberg (1956) has stated 10 activities for which the consultant has responsibility:

1. Meeting the group's initial expectations, within limits, even when their expectations do not coincide with her ideas.

2. Adjusting her own thinking to the group's approach in order to gain their confidence and help them solve their problems.

3. Giving them support when they become confused about the different aspects of the problem and presenting basic facts regarding the problem.

4. Assuring the group that their ideas are sound and worthwhile and making them feel relatively free from criticism.

5. Helping them to understand what their problem really is and what stage of problem solving they are in.

6. Helping them define their problem when they are vaguely aware that they have one but are unable to focus their thinking on its crucial aspects.

7. Using her own knowledge of nursing and her broad understanding of their problems to clear away any fuzziness in their thinking so that they may direct their own ideas toward the most important aspect of the problem.

8. Helping them to see what role they play in the project, especially when they "cannot see the forest for the trees."

9. Aiding them in evaluating the facts so they understand how the problem affects their responsibilities.

10. Making plans with the group for solving their problem and applying problem-solving methods.

The use of these activities may help the CNS to further understand the consultant role and also keep it (the role) within the limits of consultation.

There are a number of areas to be discussed when attempting to implement a consultative process. These include management support, credibility with staff, mechanisms for referral, limitations, and problem-solving skills. Each of these areas needs to be discussed separately. Management support must be sought and gained at all levels if the CNS is to be successful at consultation. The CNS should utilize all of her interpersonal techniques to gain management support for consultation by nurses. The head nurse can be a valuable ally or the downfall for the CNS's consultative efforts. Discussing the process of consultation may help her to raise questions she may have about that process. Encouraging the head nurse in her own consultative efforts adds yet another person who can be used by staff nurses as a role model for consultation. Not only the head nurse but also the director of nursing and other administrative persons must lend support to consultation by nurses. This support can usually be gained by keeping management informed about the CNS's plans for consultation. The CNS must remember that advanced practice indicates there is a right and responsibility to consult with nurses and other health care professionals about nursing care matters.

Credibility of the CNS must be perceived by the staff nurses if they are to use her as an expert consultant. The CNS cannot expect to be asked to consult if she is not seen as having specific expertise in an area. If the CNS has implemented the roles of teacher, practitioner, and researcher, it is more likely that she will be seen as the expert. This would indicate that it may take a year or longer for the CNS to be routinely involved in consultation. Consultation is difficult to implement if there are no mechanisms available to aid its implementation. Established lines for consultation may already be in place when the CNS arrives. If so, the CNS should strive to support those lines while trying to open new lines. If there are no consultative lines, the CNS can develop them by using various health care professionals as consultants. For example, a CNS working in a pediatric unit might seek out a surgical CNS to consult in problems a child may have after an operation. This will develop a network of people who will tend to use each other for consultation and who can serve as role models for the staff nurses. Because documentation is essential to good practice, most hospitals have a form that is used by all health professionals in obtaining consults. It may be best for the CNS to use already established forms so that it will be easier for staff nurses to "order" a consultation. If no such form is available, the CNS may need to design one (see Figure 7.2).

There are, of course, certain limitations to one's consultative abilities. Caplan (1970, p. 93) states that "the consultant . . . must have three aspects of functioning in reaction to the consultee—empathy, tolerance of feelings and the conviction that with enough information, all human behavior is understandable." This statement by Caplan presents some of the limitations to consultation, in particular, obtaining enough information. It is frequently difficult to obtain the amount of information to adequately assess the situation—seeing "both sides of the coin" as it were. The CNS can deal with this by taking adequate time and not rushing to make recommendations. It is better to take longer than to make inappropriate recommendations, which may then lead staff to not see the CNS as expert. Even worse, the staff may act on those hastily derived recommendations with less than desired results. Perhaps the greatest limitation deals with what is possible. The consultant must be realistic with herself and is responsible to the consultee for presenting *realistic* recommendations. Sometimes the realities of the situation will cause the consultant to recommend solutions that are not easy for the consultee to understand. If this occurs, the consultant should make every effort to go back over the recommendations presented with further explanations and time for questions. Yet another set of limitations may lie within the consultant herself. She may at times use her power to improperly influence the consultee to her way of thinking. When this approach is used, the consultee feels a loss of power over the situation and may hesitate to consult with that person again. The consultant, in an effort to gain an "in" with the consultee, may promise more than she can deliver. If this occurs, the consultee is likely to lose trust

NURSE CONSULTATION

PATIENT _____ DATE _____

UNIT _____

REASON FOR CONSULTATION _____

_____

_____

SIGNATURE _____

_____

CONSULTANT REPORT

_____

_____

_____

_____

_____

_____

_____

_____

_____

_____

_____

_____

_____

_____

_____

_____

_____

_____

_____

_____

_____

_____

_____

_____

_____

_____

_____

_____

_____

_____

_____

_____

_____

_____

_____

_____

SIGNATURE _____

Figure 7.2. Nurse Consultation form.

in the CNS, which may jeopardize future consultations. The CNS consultant, although the expert, must assume that the consultee is capable of making decisions to solve problems. The CNS should not be patronizing or try to implement a change without involving the consultee.

A major role of the CNS consultant is to help develop and refine the problem-solving skills of the consultee(s). Although the staff nurses may have knowledge of process, at times they are too involved in the situation to be able to adequately use that process without some help. The consultant is not there to solve the problem but to help the consultee to problem solve. Norris (1977) states that "it is important to keep clarifying who does the work and who resolves the problem." If the CNS keeps this at the forefront, she is less likely to be trapped into handling the entire problem herself. Stevens (1978, p. 13) has written that most groups' interactions with a consultant go through four stages: a time for thoroughly discussing all aspects of the situation, or "cathexis, the search for a 'quick cure,' acceptance of the need for internal work, and the search for real problems and solutions." By knowing these stages, the CNS can better assist the consultee(s) to problem solve. It will be very difficult during the first two stages to do any of the real work of problem solving, but a failure to recognize this may lead to discouragement with the consulting process. The CNS must understand and assist the consultee(s) through these two stages so that productive problem solving can begin.

One final aspect of consultation for the CNS is that which is done for a fee. The CNS may find that her expertise is marketable as a consultant. Nuckolls (1977) offers some guidelines for the consultant in the form of questions. They include (p. 14):

1) How well defined is the client's problem? 2) Is this a sincere request? 3) Is the problem in your field of competence: 4) Is it short or long term? 5) How much time commitment is needed? 6) Can you get time off from your regular job? 7) May you accept a fee? 8) Is there a conflict of interest? 9) Do you really want to do this?

When these questions have been answered and the consultation is accepted, a fee must be negotiated and expectations agreed upon. With these initial steps in place, one then proceeds with the consultation process.

The preceding practical points are offered to help the CNS begin consulting. The following discussion using the steps in consultation may help to further clarify the consultation process. A case study will follow this chapter delineating how one CNS utilized the consultative role.

CLINICAL SITUATION

Consultative Step	Discussion
I. Request: The CNS for a pediatric intensive care unit was consulted by the staff as they began to prepare an orientation for new nurses to the unit. They were specifically asking for help in the type of orientation to use and what to include in the orientation.	The CNS gained entry when the nurses asked for help in preparing an orientation. At this point, it would have been an easy mistake for the CNS to take over the entire project.
II. Diagnosis: The CNS looked at various types of models for orientation, including one that a graduate student had suggested. These were shown to the staff. Additionally, the CNS collected information of differing levels on common procedures in the unit. The staff looked at all of the information and gave their comments. Based on all of the data, the CNS was able to make an assessment of the particular type of orientation needed and the content for the orientation.	An appropriate diagnosis could only be made if the CNS took the time needed to look at all aspects of various orientation models. Making a diagnosis too quickly can result in the wrong recommendations.
III. Planned Action: After diagnosing the needs of the group, the CNS made her recommendations. She felt that the model suggested by the graduate student best filled the orientation needs as well as the staff's philosophy. She also made recommendations on content to be included in the orientation. The staff found that the	The staff chose to accept most of the recommendations of the consultant. Had they decided not to accept, the CNS could have closed the consultation after an evaluation or she could have presented additional recommendations after further study.

CLINICAL SITUATION

Consultative Step	Discussion
suggested model did seem to fit their needs. The CNS also recommended that the graduate student assist the staff to organize the orientation. This recommendation was also accepted by the staff. The CNS documented her findings on a consultant's report.	
IV. Evaluation: After the project recommendations had been made, accepted and implemented, the CNS held a conference with the staff to determine if they felt comfortable with the orientation. The staff expressed satisfaction and were sure they could work out any remaining problems in the orientation.	The evaluative period gave the staff the chance to verbalize how they saw the orientation process. It was also another opportunity for the CNS to answer any further questions the staff might have.
V. Closure: The CNS stated that since the staff was comfortable with the orientation, she would be available at any time for questions but that they should continue the excellent job they were doing.	In closing, the CNS acknowledged that the staff was exceedingly capable in handling the orientation. She also gave them an opportunity to call for more help as needed. Additionally, the CNS should follow closure with a phone call or visit to the staff to allow further consultation if needed.

BIBLIOGRAPHY

Abramovitz, A. (1958). Methods and techniques of consultation. *American Journal of Orthopsychiatry*, **28**, 126–133.

Ashworth, P. (1976, May 13). The role of the clinical nurse consultant. *Nursing Mirror*, **20**(142), 46–48.

Belko, P., & Menard, S. (1982, April). The PICU: A model for orientation. *Nursing Management,* **14**(4), 36–37.

Blake, P. (1977, December). The clinical specialist as nurse consultant. *Journal of Nursing Administration*, **7**(10), 33–36.

Blount, M., Burge, S., Crigler, L., Finkelmeier, B., & Samborn, C. (1981, Fall). Extending the influence of the clinical nurse specialist. *Nursing Administration Quarterly*, **6**(1), 53–63.

Blumberg, A., (1956, May). A nurse consultant's responsibility and problems. *American Journal of Nursing*, **56**(3), 606–698.

Boehm, W. (1956). The professional relationship between consultant and consultee. *American Journal of Orthopsychiatry*, **26**, 241–248.

Caplan, G. (1970). *The theory and practice of mental health consultation.* New York: Basic Books.

Evans, D. & Sutton, G. (1973, December). A case for consultation. *Nursing Clinics of North America*, **8**(4), 751–756.

Kohnke, M. (1978). *Case for consultation in nursing: Designs for professional practice.* (pp. 55–83). New York: Wiley.

Norris, C. (1977, December). A few notes on consultation in nursing. *Nursing Outlook*, **77**(12), 756–761.

Norton, L. (1981, Fall). The clinical nurse specialist as consultant. *Nursing Administration Quarterly*, **6**(1), 69–75.

Nuckolls, K. (1977, January/February). The consultation process: A reciprocal relationship. *Maternal Child Nursing*, **2**(1), 11–16.

Sedgwick, R. (1973, December). The role of the process consultant. *Nursing Outlook*, **21**(12), 773–775.

Stevens, B.J. (1978, August). The use of consultants in nursing practice. *Journal of Nursing Administration,* **8**(8), 7–15.

Termini, M. & Ciechoski, M. (1981) The consultation process. *Issues in Mental Health Nursing*, **3**, 77–88.

Will, M. (1977, December). Referral: A process, not a form. *Nursing '77*, 44–45.

CASE STUDY: ESTABLISHING THE CNS CONSULTANT ROLE
Susan Cooning, M.S., R.N.

Establishing the consultant role can be a challenge. While eventually nurses may learn to make referrals to the nurse specialist, many of my CNS colleagues report that they experience some problem in being accepted as a legitimate consultant by physicians. As Nurse Coordinator of Children's Hospital new Nutrition Support Service (NSS), I found physician utilization of my services came more readily than did nursing utilization. However, even though physicians requested my services to perform central line dressing changes, this was due more to a need to provide special "technology" to the patient rather than an indicator that the physician understood and accepted the CNS role. But it was by providing a technological service for the patient and then expanding the "skill" of dressing changes to include troubleshooting with problems the patient might develop, such as skin breakdown and site infection, that led to an increased acceptance of my role by physicians. Eventually, I gained enough credibility with physicians that my recommendation to culture or discontinue a central line based on nursing observation of symptoms of infection at the site or to increase IV carbohydrate due to poor weight gain were more readily accepted.

In my CNS role I was a member of a multidisciplinary team that included a gastroenterologist, surgeon, pharmacist, clinical nutritionist, and nurse IV therapists. The apparent "acceptance" of my CNS role by staff physicians was more related to my association with other physician team members than true understanding of the CNS role. The nurse specialist must be aware that being viewed by physicians as "Dr. G's nurse" does not indicate an understanding of the true scope of the CNS role. I had to continually work to correct this physician perception and avoid being labeled as another doctor's nurse by always providing more than just the technical skill of changing central line dressings in an aseptic manner. I continued to monitor and document patient response to nutrition therapy such as changes in laboratory findings and weight changes and to make recommendations for therapy changes based on my clinical observations. I also responded to patient and family learning needs as part of my CNS role, documenting teaching and discharge planning in the same progress notes used by physicians as did other specialists. After about a 9-month "initiation" period, physicians began to request CNS input into nutritional assessment and ongoing monitoring, family and patient teaching, and home care planning. Nurses were quicker than physicians to accept me in my expanded role, but I first had to "prove" myself as a provider of a specialized technological skill such as central line dressing changes. Nurses learned that when a patient problem related to delivery of hyperalimentation and central lines occurred as well as when patient behavior changes such as lethargy and weakness became apparent, I could be counted on to respond to the nurses' request for consultation. Some of the strategies we used to gain credibility and acceptance as a team could also be of benefit to the CNS in establishing the consultant role.

USE OF A CONSULTANT REQUEST FORM

One of the most helpful tools in developing my CNS consultant role was a consultant request form. Although this form was developed by the NSS, there was space for the nurse or physician requesting the consult to indicate the services desired, such as comprehensive nutritional assessment, calorie count, central line dressing change, or home care planning. Not only did the form provide a brief list of services provided by the NSS but there was also space for a report of consultation. The original consult form remained a part of the patient's medical record, and a copy was kept in NSS files for billing and recordkeeping purposes. The CNS could develop a similar form, listing services such as diabetic instruction and discharge planning, to clearly identify areas of expertise.

In developing my consultant role, I learned that an immediate response to a referral was vital even though I might be notified of a new consultation request at 5 P.M. on a Friday afternoon. In my initial report, I found it helpful to provide a written assessment of the patient and the clinical situation along with an outline of the plan. In situations where continued follow-up was required, I used the same format in the progress notes. I quickly learned that when making recommendations for further testing or for enteral formula changes that required a physician's order, physician follow-up was more likely when I offered written rationale for my recommendation and then communicated in person with the referring physician. The CNS who makes recommendations for therapy changes based on clinical judgment is often perceived as threatening by physicians.

When acting on a nursing referral, I outlined my assessment and plan in the progress notes to inform medical staff and other consultants of my involvement. A summary in the nurses notes and on the patient care plan was the best mechanism to communicate with nurses. Often the nursing referrals I received as a NSS team member required central line dressing changes. Initially, I performed these dressing changes myself, and later, the nurse IV therapist had this responsibility. The IV therapy nurse, also part of the NSS, documented dressing changes and condition of the IV site in the medical progress notes.

LIMITATIONS IN THE CONSULTANT ROLE

As a new CNS, I found it important to learn the limitations of my consultant role. The nurse consultant makes suggestions and provides a rationale when responding to a medical referral. The physician may choose a different course of action other than what the CNS recommends. With nursing referrals, it was important for me as the CNS to problem solve *with* nursing staff, not *for* the nursing staff. My ultimate goal as a CNS is to promote independence of the patient and family and to promote independence and problem solving by the nursing staff. The CNS role should not be to develop and write the care plan alone and deliver the specialized nursing care single-handedly. Nursing staff need to be involved and to maintain a major role in the development of the plan and in the delivery of care. There were many times early in my CNS role development when nursing relinquished responsibility for nursing invervention with a patient who had complex psychosocial needs. Physical needs were met, but the psychosocial and teaching needs were sometimes "dumped" on the CNS. The important thing in these cases was to focus on patient needs and outcomes. Often nursing "territory" had to be hashed out after the fact, and often I did deal with the patient needs that nursing staff felt ill-equipped or too overwhelmed to deal with. By identifying the areas nursing staff felt uncomfortable dealing with and then working with them to improve in those areas, these situations occurred less and less frequently.

Often response to a nursing referral meant becoming involved in the medical care of the patient. For example, nurses requesting my assistance in monitoring a peripheral IV line in a child often led to a recommendation to the physician for central line placement. Nurses began to learn through CNS examples that with appropriate documentation and rationale, they too could approach the physician with the recommendation for a central line without the CNS running interference. This was a great step forward for nursing staff, and the ability to make such recommendations evolved over a long period of time.

PROMOTING STAFF NURSING INDEPENDENCE

At times, I would receive a nursing referral on a patient problem that really required a medical referral and intervention. I still responded to the referral, but often my recommendation was to notify the appropriate physician. I think nurses sometimes used me in my CNS consultant role just to validate what they already knew needed to be done. But even inappropriate referrals initially served to open the door for me to become more involved as a CNS in the coordination of nursing care for many patients I otherwise would never have seen.

In other instances, the nurse might call me to verify that a certain patient situation warranted physician intervention or was indeed an emergency situation. As nurses gained more self-confidence in their own judgment, inappropriate CNS referrals became less frequent. As nurses became more informed as to my areas of nursing expertise and learned to trust my recommendations, referrals from nursing came more frequently.

USE OF THE CARE CONFERENCE IN THE CONSULTANT ROLE

When our NSS service received a referral for discharge planning for a patient with complex nutrition needs, as NSS nurse coordinator my responsibility was to set up a discharge planning conference. This involved NSS team members as well as other relevant physicians, nurses, social workers, and home care representatives.

In addition to my NSS role, I still had responsibilities to serve as a CNS consultant for nursing service. In this role, I also found myself responsible for identifying the need for a patient conference in order to coordinate the complex care of a particular patient. As a CNS consultant, as well as in my NSS nurse consultant role, I would often be the person to plan the conference time and place and to invite members from appropriate disciplines. I learned to clearly state the goals and expectations for the conference as I invited each participant. Before convening the conference, everyone involved had to be informed as to its focus — whether our purpose was to develop a discharge plan, revise the nursing plan of care, or plan an approach to deal effectively with an unstable family situation. Sometimes I found it helpful to "prime" certain individuals as to what to bring out in the conference. For example, if the patient needed a primary nurse, I would try to meet with the head nurse prior to the conference in order to identify the most appropriate nurse to meet the patient and/or family needs. If the goal of the conference was to develop a consistent approach in discipline for a hospitalized child, the staff psychologist would be invited to attend the conference and bring a discipline plan appropriate for that particular child.

Usually the person calling the conference was responsible for taking notes. Later we developed a system of rotating note-taking responsibilities among all team members. This required developing a format for recording the minutes of a care conference to ensure that information such as the concerns discussed, goals developed, and persons responsible for follow-up of each goal would be clearly stated. The conference minutes were typed and became a part of the patient's permanent medical record.

As a CNS, I often had sole responsibility for coordinating patient care conferences. In my NSS role, this was a consultant service provided by our team for which I was responsible as nurse coordinator. In my CNS consultant role for nursing service, care conferences were not to be only my responsibility, but initially it was necessary for me to serve as a nursing role model. Later individual nurses would assume responsibility for setting up care conferences, or often a child life worker or social worker would initiate the conference. One goal that was never realized was for a physician to be the initiator and coordinator of a patient care conference.

The reason care conferences are emphasized here is because they assisted me in identifying my CNS role to other disciplines, and it demonstrated my willingness to work with and follow up on difficult patient situations. The care conference was probably one of the most valuable avenues for increasing CNS involvement in patient care. Previous to my implementing the first CNS role in this hospital, care conferences were used very infrequently to plan and coordinate patient care. Although patient care conferences certainly were not a new concept, they increased in frequency and productivity after my arrival in the CNS role. The care conference was therefore seen as "my" contribution to improving the delivery and coordination of nursing care.

The other very valuable result of the care conference was that goals were developed using a team approach, and care was not just "planned" by the CNS. When responsibilities were assigned to individuals in the presence of co-workers from other disciplines, pressure to follow through was applied by team members, not by the nurse specialist. In this way, care conferences provided a mechanism for assigning responsibility as well as for individual acceptance of that responsibility.

In addition to the consult form and the patient care conference, another method that helped me establish my CNS consultant role was to attend morning report in the nursing supervisors' office. An exchange of information between the night shift supervisors and the day shift supervisors not only clued me in to such things as hospitalwide patient census and staffing shortages but also gave me an update on new patients, patients with new central lines, and unusual occurrences or problems concerning nursing care of patients. By being present at report every morning, I could get nursing referrals from the supervisors or at least find out what nursing unit might require CNS services. At times I had to actively solicit referrals with the head nurses in order to get involved with a patient with complex nursing care needs. Sometimes, based on information received in morning report, I could identify nursing continuing education needs on a unit-by-unit basis and either develop an inservice or collaborate with the Department of Nursing Education to meet specific educational needs.

An avenue I also found helpful in soliciting nursing referrals was to accompany the head nurses on patient rounds whenever possible. Often, I could offer suggestions or provide alternatives that assisted nurses in meeting patient and family needs. This type of informal involvement often led to formal nursing referrals.

Another mechanism utilized in publicizing the NSS and its team members that I have since found helpful in introducing a new CNS role is the hospital media department. Our hospital's Department of Communications interviewed each NSS team member and described our individual roles as well as team goals and services for the hospital newspaper. Pictures were included to identify not only each team member but also some of the long-term nutrition patients we worked with. A similar report on the NSS concept appeared in the hospital's annual report publication.

After about a year of NSS operation as a team, one of our patients attracted local media attention because of his youth and his dependency on IV nutrition. Once again, our service and its members were highlighted in a detailed report of this child's medical condition and "miracle" survival. Individual interviews and scenes of the child's hospital environment presented on the six o'clock television news informed the public of the child's critical needs and the specific services provided him by NSS. This example may seem rather extreme, but media focus on a particular patient almost always includes aspects of his nursing care requirements along with the nursing care providers.

The CNS can utilize any or all of the methods discussed in establishing credibility as a consultant. It is always necessary to tailor these methods to fit the setting, but I have been able to use many of the same methods to make myself known and increase CNS visibility in subsequent CNS roles I have had to develop. My experience has shown that it takes time to forge a new role. Anywhere from 6 months to a year has passed in some settings before I have been able to identify progress in role identification. It helps to identify institutional and nursing needs. To formulate a plan, set realistic goals, identify support people, and assertively develop your CNS role. A plan of evaluation can also help demonstrate definite progress toward role definition and refinement when the nurse specialist may believe there is none on a day-to-day basis.

8

THE CNS AS RESEARCHER

Joan M. Wabschall, M.S., R.N.

Chapter Objectives

At the conclusion of this chapter, the reader will:

1. Describe the relationship between science and nursing research.
2. Identify nursing activities other than formal research that the clinical nurse specialist (CNS) can participate in to develop research process skills.
3. Differentiate between nursing research and research in nursing.
4. Systematically evaluate the research climate within the practice setting.
5. Identify strategies that will facilitate the introduction and implementation of nursing research within an institution.
6. Identify nursing groups that are available to lend support to the CNS in research efforts.
7. Examine personal values and commitment to the research role.

Early in the history of the utilization of clinical nurse specialists (CNSs), the profession looked to the CNS as the professional who would advance the science of nursing by being an expert role model in the clinical setting and by commitment to systematically investigating problems and concerns in the practice of nursing. With advanced preparation at the master's level, these nurses were viewed as critical thinkers and as nurses who would make an impact on patient outcome by their demonstrated excellence in practice.

While administrators may not overly acknowledge the CNS's role in research, a review of job descriptions would reveal the concepts of research that are incorporated in the CNS role. For example, phrases such as "uses sytematic methods of scientific inquiry to investigate patient care and nursing problems," "supports and encourages the spirit of inquiry in others," and "applies a theoretical framework as a rationale for practice" all connote the process used in nursing research even though the word *research* is not mentioned. The key phrases here are "systematic methods," "application of a theoretical framework," and "scientific inquiry." CNSs should be able to incorporate these concepts into their daily use of the nursing process and facilitate an atmosphere of support for systematic observation and planned interventions by staff nurses.

With all the demands placed on the CNS in the roles of expert clinician, administrator, educator, and consultant, it is not surprising that research activities are often a low priority for the CNS. Conducting formal research in a service setting can be a very time-consuming effort, especially if the atmosphere for acceptance of nursing research has not been established. However, CNSs are in a unique position to facilitate nursing research because of their level of knowledge and commitment to clinical practice.

Hinshaw, Chance, and Atwood (1981) believe that the focus of a clinically oriented nurse is on the relevancy of research to the practice situation, while the focus of the nurse researcher is on precision and accuracy of data collection in the investigation of a research problem. They state (p. 34): "The knowledge, skills, and priorities of both clinician and researcher can be merged, with each protecting the integrity of his or her view of the project." The CNS is the logical person to integrate the dual roles of clinician and researcher and thus become a nurse scientist. When given the administrative support and professional encouragement, the CNS who is committed to research can accomplish great feats in an institution where nursing research is an expected part of clinical practice.

The development of the science of nursing is a professional responsibility of all nurses. The CNS can take a leadership role in that development. Research has been the foundation of many recognized sciences. It is only with the marriage of nursing practice and a questioning mind that the science of nursing can advance to a point where even the public is convinced that nurses make a difference in patient care. Who is better suited to make an impact on the practice of nursing through research than the CNS?

While few professionals will argue the need for nursing research to better define the practice of nursing, a number of controversies surface when one examines the nursing profession as a science. In this chapter, we will study some of the unsettled questions in the development of the science of nursing and examine the role of the CNS in advancing the profession through nursing research. The focus of the CNS's involvement with research, however, will be approached from the perspective of how to incorporate various levels of nursing research into the role rather than the specifics of how to design and conduct a scientific study. The intent is to expose the reader to a variety of thought-provoking concepts and to give practical strategies on how the CNS can promote research within a service setting.

THE NATURE OF SCIENCE

The results of science and technology have a profound impact on society. Science is a way of knowing, and research is the method of generating that new knowledge or the relationships that exist between that which is being studied. Science and research in science has influenced, and will continue to influence, our every-day life.

If we analyze common definitions of science, we find terminology that is not all that foreign to the practice of nursing. Observation is a key component in science. It is through the scientific method of observation and experimentation that new knowledge is derived. Classification is a way of organizing knowledge into groupings within the discipline being studied so that the knowledge is more easily understood by others. Verification of phenomena relates to the ability of science to be confirmed by repeated observations and experimentation. The term *empirical* is often used to refer to the same concept as verification. Nursing is clearly involved with observation, classification, and verification. For instance, nursing involves the observation of other humans during health or illness, classifies observations into planned interventions, and verifies, validates, and evaluates the care given. Since nursing uses all the major activites of science, it can legitimately be called a science.

The building blocks of scientific thought are numerous. They include observations that lead to facts, which in turn help to identify concepts. Concepts generate theories that require testing and eventually lead to scientific laws that govern our universe (Bush, 1985). When the starting point for the development of science is at the observational level and proceeds up the ladder as described above, the process is referred to as inductive reasoning. If, on the other hand, one begins with a higher level on the ladder (laws or theories, for example) and works down to test the applicability of the laws or theories on the observational level, the process is referred to as deductive reasoning (see Figure 8.1).

Both inductive and deductive reasoning are valuable components of systematic study. Nurses who identify problems in nursing practice while giving

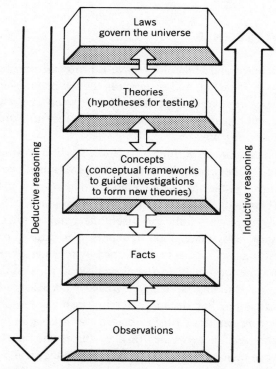

Figure 8.1. Building blocks of scientific thought. (From *Bush, C.T., Building Block of Scientific Thought, Reston, WV, Reston Publishing, 1985. Permission granted.*)

patient care will utilize inductive principles of scientific inquiry while they study the phenomenon. By contrast, an example of deductive reasoning is the nurse's utilization of Orem's self-care theory to teach postoperative care in a day surgery unit and the conduct of a study to document the retention of learning under those conditions. One method of reasoning is not superior to another. It is the situation in which the nursing care takes place that will determine the appropriateness of the method to be used in building scientific thought.

Inductive and deductive reasoning are methods of research. Cormack (1984, p. 4) defines research as "an attempt to increase the sum of what is known . . . by the discovery of new facts of relationships through a process of systematic scientific inquiry, the research process." The research process is preplanned and carried out to test observations that will lead to a new body of knowledge.

The new knowledge that is generated through research can be divided into two categories: basic and applied science. Using Johnson's definition (cited in Fox & Leeser, 1981) of these two types of science, one finds a difference in the philosophical natures of basic and applied sciences. Basic science is committed to the task of explaining natural phenomena by scientific investigation and to the systematization of knowledge. By contrast, applied science draws heavily on the basic sciences to derive another body of knowledge and is committed to the application of knowledge toward some well-defined social goal. Nursing is being recognized increasingly as a science, but the dilemma continues as to whether nursing is an applied or a basic science.

PROFESSIONAL NURSING AS A SCIENCE

The history of nursing education reveals that a variety of sciences have been utilized as a background for the teaching of nursing: microbiology, chemistry, nutrition, anatomy, physiology, pharmacology, psychology, sociology, and even philosophy. Some of these disciplines are basic sciences, and others are considered humanities. Concepts from these other disciplines have been borrowed to formulate nursing concepts. For this reason, many believe that nursing is an applied science.

Johnson's article (cited in Fox & Lessor, 1981) is a strong argument for defining nursing as an applied science. She contends that nursing has as its ultimate goal the promotion and maintenance of optimal health for individuals and for groups. This is a social goal that nursing shares with other health workers. Nursing is an applied science, according to Johnson, because it is committed to the task of utilizing knowledge to achieve this well-defined social goal.

Wald and Leonard (also cited in Fox & Leeser, 1981) can be considered opponents of the Johnson viewpoint. They believe that no matter how much principles borrowed from the basic sciences are accepted as pure science, the same principles may be invalid or inappropriate when used in the nursing situation. The fact that many of these borrowed concepts have not been tested in the clinical nursing setting only further implies the need for establishing principles, based on research, that can become the foundation of nursing practice.

The practice of pursuing nursing knowledge through the untested application of principles from the social sciences is a major concern of Wald and Leonard (cited in Fox & Leeser, 1981). They believe that nurses have rephrased nursing problems as social science questions rather than as questions of nursing practice. An alternative to this method of building nursing theory from applied science is to begin with practical nursing experience and inductively develop concepts from an analysis of the clinical experience rather than by trying to make borrowed concepts from other sciences fit the nursing situation. Kerlinger (1977) proposes that there has been an overemphasis on applied research within professions and supports the opinion that basic research has greater impact on practice than applied research.

Although applied and basic sciences have their differences, there are also many similarities between them. Both are concerned with a connected body of truths, both utilize the scientific method and contribute to increasing the world's knowledge, and both have social values (Johnson, cited in Fox & Leeser, 1981). The argument to determine where nursing fits within the sciences will continue as the profession matures. It is philosophical arguments such as this that will encourage nurses to think for themselves and to exercise judgment in scientific thought.

Methods of Nursing Research: Quantitative versus Qualitative

Not only are we uncertain whether nursing is an applied or a basic science but there is also debate as to the methods of research that best describe what nursing is all about. Quantitative methods rely heavily on mathematics as the language of science. This method of research measures variables and demonstrates findings in terms of amounts (Cormack, 1984). Qualitative research, on the other hand, is based on the premise that there is more to knowing people than what can be seen, sensed, and measured. (For a complete contrast between quantitative and qualitative methodologies, see Table 8.1.)

The profession of nursing has probably relied upon quantitative methods of research more frequently than qualitative methods because of nursing's relative newness to the world of research. In order to gain equal footing with the other professions, the language of mathematics has been employed to legitimize the research being conducted by nurses. Americans have been traditionally influenced by the early European culture in which the scientific movement began. Western culture has long believed that there is a single scientific method and that science has nothing to say about value (Leininger, 1985).

Additional reasons why qualitative research has been a latecomer on the research scene have been related to the lack of knowledge in qualitative research methods on the part of nurse educators. By not being well versed in these methods, nursing faculty have perpetuated acceptance of the quantitative methodologies as the "only" research that would be regarded as scientific. Qualitative research does not get funded as frequently, nor is it accepted for publication as often as quantitative research (Leininger, 1985).

When one adheres to the definition of nursing as published in the ANA Social Policy Statement (1980), nursing is a science that formulates the diagnosis and treatment of human responses to actual or potential health problems. Human care is the critical and essential element of nursing. Leininger (1984, p. xi) states:

> Humanistic and scientific components of care require quite different research methods and modes of analysis than quantitative methods of data collection and analysis. To discover the nature of human care necessitates exquisite participant observations, interviews, documentations, and other research skills and techniques associated with qualitative types of research.

It is beyond the scope of this chapter to outline the various forms of qualitative studies. However, the CNS needs to keep in mind that both quantitative and qualitative methods provide valuable frameworks for research. The crucial point is to know when to use each type.

Table 8.1. Contrasts of Qualitative and Quantitative Methodologies

Domains	Qualitative Methodology	Quantitative Methodology
Definitional focus	Nature, essence, meaning, and attributes (what it is and characteristics); teleological	Measurement focus of a thing, object, or subject (how much)
General research focus	Description, documentation, and analysis of patterns, values, essences, world view, meanings, beliefs, and attitudes; totality of experiences in natural or particular contexts	Measurement of controlled or manipulated variables by experimental, quasi-experimental, and other controlled methods; causal and measurable relationships
Scope	Generally broad, holistic, and comprehensive; world view; includes more than excludes phenomena to know totality aspects	Particularist, narrow, and limited focus; controlled; excludes more than includes
Setting	Naturalistic and generally familiar setting where life patterning frequently occurs	Often unfamiliar laboratory or artificial settings to control and manipulate variables
Orientation	Process and phenomena oriented; open discovery, exploratory, comparative, expanding, inclusive, and descriptive; Usually inductive and emic discovery approach; Local viewpoints emphasized	Outcome or product oriented; Generally a closed, narrowly defined, and restricted approach; oriented to reduction and manipulation of control variables; Deductively oriented
Research goal	Development of understandings and meanings of what one sees, hears, experiences, and discovers through a variety of sensual observation–participation modes; obtain a full and accurate "truth" from people	Testing hypotheses to obtain measurable outcomes among variables under study; precision and objective findings

Table 8.1. *Continued*

Domains	Qualitative Methodology	Quantitative Methodology
Relation to people being studied	Frequently direct involvement and participation with people	Generally noninvolvement, nonparticipation, and detachment from subjects
Root source of knowledge	Cultural (ethnography), social, environmental, and philosophical phenomena to obtain patterned human interactions, symbols, values, world views, historical and general ethnographic lifeways	Logical positivism, with use of human senses; Psychological and biophysical facts and causes of things, objects, or behaviors; empiricism valued
Data sought	Seek subjective and objective data; inclusive	Seek mainly objective data; exclusive
Study focus	Participants, informants, role takers, respondents, and people	Objects, subjects, cases, data banks, code numbers, and figures
Domains of analysis	Can reformulate and expand focus of study as one proceeds; no predetermined and no "a priori" judgments; open discovery; flexible and dynamic; moves with people, context, situation, or events	Predetermined; a fixed design; prejudgments and "a priori" position taken; rigid and fixed categories; nondynamic; fixed and planned sequence of research design to reduce variances;
"Tools" for investigation	The instrument is mainly the researcher; uses field study tools as observation guides, open-ended interviews, direct participation, documents, open frames, guides, life histories, audiovisual media, biographies, diaries, kingrams, and many other tools	Questionnaires, surveys, and special tools to control variables, highly structured interviews, and an array of precise tools to elicit precise responses; computer is a major tool

Table 8.1. *Continued*

Domains	Qualitative Methodology	Quantitative Methodology
Modes of analysis	Content, symbolic, structural, interactional, philosophical, ethnographic, semantic, historical, inferential, perceptual, and reflexive types of analysis; diverse and creative modes of analysis to fit context and purposes of research; diverse qualitative approaches	Various statistical analysis methods; predetermined data sets; must use only what has been collected; regressive, experimental, and survey analysis; largely computer analyzed; inputs and outputs
Validity indicators	"Truth" as known to the people; understandings, insight, accuracy, confirmation, completeness of information; the people's viewpoints or world view (emic) is mainly sought; a few etic inferences for truths	Statistical significance, alpha-beta levels, measurable, "hard" proof and objective measurements; internal and external measurable validity factors
Reliability indicators	Recurrent themes, patterns, life-styles, and behaviors; historical and time context, single or small group special features; difficult to replicate due to unique aspects of context in time and space	Repeated measures, generalizable to other "cases"; data can be generalized or repeated for large groups; reproducibility
Problem areas	large amount of qualitative data to analyze	Defined, controlled, and selected quantifiable data to analyze

From Leininger, M., *Contrasts of Qualitative and Quantitative Methodologies*, Orlando, FL, Grune & Stratton, 1985. Permission granted.

Problem Solving as a Basis for Nursing

Exercises in problem solving have been a part of professional nursing for years. Patient care is fraught with problems that require nursing assessment, planned intervention, and evaluation. Think for a moment of the patient whose IV is not infusing properly. The nurse assesses the site, investigates the delivery system of the infusate, makes an adjustment, and then evaluates the outcome. Whether the IV line is patent and only needs a new bottle of fluid hung or whether the IV has infiltrated the patient's tissue, the decision to keep the IV in place or to discontinue it is an example of problem solving in nursing practice.

The process of problem solving involves three basic questions and brings to mind the steps of the nursing process:

1. What is the problem?
2. How are solutions sought?
3. Do the answers resolve the problem?

Padilla (1979) describes a continuum of patient care evaluation that has the nursing process as the most basic form of problem solving and nursing research as the most sophisticated method of problem solving. The two processes in between are the problem-oriented medical record (POMR) and the nursing audit. All four of the processes address the same basic questions. For a contrast of these four processes, see Figure 8.2.

The POMR includes a systematic method of assessing the patient and a standardized format for documentation. Problems are listed succinctly. While POMR deals with multiple problems, it allows a basic application of the research framework (Padilla, 1979).

Quality assurance methods comprise the next level of sophistication within the patient care evaluation continuum. Quality assurance efforts are more similar to nursing research than the other two levels because they focus on groups of patients much as the research process studies populations. Quality assurance criteria should be grounded in the best available science, which becomes available through the development of nursing research (Bloch, 1980).

Nurses, in general, are familiar with the nursing process, with POMR,

Basic Questions For Problem Solving	Nursing Process	Problem-Oriented Medical Record	Nursing Audit	Nursing Research
			Select Population	
			Determine Outcome Criteria	
What is the problem/ question?	Assess patient status	Define data base Historical, demographic data Physiological data Laboratory data	Audit outcome criteria	Evaluate preliminary data Pilot study/ audit of outcome criteria/ clinical experiences
				Define problem and population
	Define problem	List problems	Analyze audit findings Identify deficiencies	
What and how are solutions/ answers sought?	Plan intervention	Identify plans Diagnostic plan Therapeutic plan Education plan	Select corrective intervention	Review literature Select framework State hypothesis Operationally define variables Test manipulations and tools Select design Define sample Define data collection procedure
	Implement intervention	(assumed)	Implement corrective intervention	Implement study and collect data
Do the answers resolve the problem/question?	Evaluate intervention	Evaluate progress with: Subjective patient data Objective data Assessment of status of problems Plans for continuing clinical actions	Evaluate corrective intervention	Analyze data
			Revise outcome criteria	Interpret and communicate results

Figure 8.2. Processes used for patient care evaluation. *(From Padilla, G., The Journal of Nursing Administration, Vol. 9, No. 1, 1979, pp. 44–49. Used with permission.)*

and with the nursing audit. By using these activities of the research process and going one step further to a consistent focus on one problem experienced by a group of patients, nursing research can be introduced in the practice setting.

The concept of problem solving forms the foundation for the development of nursing research. Both research and problem solving are thinking processes that do not surface automatically. Both involve observation, planning, carrying out an action, and evaluation (Trussell, Brandt, & Knapp, 1981). On the other hand, nursing research is different from problem solving in that it is more efficient, less prone to bias, more generalizable, more valid than the trial-and-error method often used in problem solving, and more objective, precise, and theory oriented than the nursing process (Stetler, 1983).

In summary, problem solving and research do have areas in common, but they also have their differences. These differences are made apparent by "the situations in which they are carried out, the conditions under which they are done, and the expertise required to do them" (Trussell, et al., 1981, p. 8). If the CNS can recognize these differences and focus on the similarities of research and the very familiar aspects of problem solving, nursing research will become a reality for more practicing nurses.

Nursing Research versus Research in Nursing

Beginning researchers find the formulation of research question difficult. With research being a rather new expectation of the professional nurse, the possibilities for research are endless. If one examines the type of research done within the profession of nursing, one learns of the distinction between nursing research and research in nursing.

The articles by Notter and Folta (cited in Gortner, 1975, p. 193) define nursing research as "the care process and the problems that are encountered in the practice of nursing: maintenance of hygiene, rest, sleep, nutrition, relief from pain or discomfort, counseling, health education, and rehabilitation." Historically, however, research in nursing has had as its subject the profession itself—its practitioners and the characteristics of their practices: utilization, costs, administration, career patterns, and educational concerns.

Years ago, Virginia Henderson (1956) published an article in *Nursing Research* that promoted the idea of research in practice. She stated that no other discipline studies the workers rather than the work. Why then do nurses believe they must study nurses rather than nursing itself?

More recently we have seen an increase in the number of practice-related research studies. This trend has increased to the point where we can now further subdivide practice research into four components: nursing research related to the science of practice, the artistry of practice, the structures needed for optimal delivery of patient care, and the tools and methods needed for assessment of practice (Gortner, cited in Downs & Fleming, 1979). The science of practice is that area concerned with the systematic identification of health problems and patient needs. The artistry of practice has an implied focus on what nurses do—the evaluation of nursing procedures and techniques. This area includes the physical as well as the interpersonal aspects of nursing care and evaluates the nursing intervention in terms of outcome. Research that includes the structures necessary for the provision of nursing care investigates the environments where nurses and patients interact. The last area of practice research is that of methodology development. In this area, valid and reliable tools are established that can be used to effectively assess and measure patient responses within the framework of nursing research. With this surge in practice-oriented research, it is not surprising that the CNS finds herself in the midst of expectations to continue the advancement of the profession through clinical nursing research.

The term *clinical* can have a number of connotative meanings. Clinical can refer to a place such as a hospital unit or it can refer to some entity of health or illness. In addition, clinical can mean having relevance to practice. If this latter definition is used, Newman (1982) contends that **all** nursing research is clinical.

In this chapter, clinical research is synonymous with nursing research and is defined as research that is oriented to the practice of nursing that can be evaluated in terms of patient outcome. Gortner (1975) says that the key words in defining clinical research are *patient* and *effect/outcome*. Bloch (1980) asserts that process and outcome need to be examined together. The whole purpose of nursing research is to confirm and expand the present body of knowledge in nursing practice and therefore improve health care for our patients.

With the evolution of nursing research, a science of nursing can be developed. As Kerlinger (1977, p. 10) states, "Science and scientific research change our ways of thinking about ourselves. . . . A profession, once thoroughly exposed to science, can never be the same."

ESSENTIAL QUALITIES OF THE NURSE SCIENTIST

The nurse researcher is a nurse scientist. Being a successful researcher and a nurse scientist requires certain qualities. First and foremost, the nurse must be a critical thinker, one who is continuously asking questions with the ultimate goal of improving nursing practice. Creativity is also essential. Nurses must exercise independence and creativity in thought in order to be true innovators in research. According to Brown (cited in Fox & Leeser, 1981, p. 16),

> the ability to think creatively differentiates the scientist from the research technologist. Order in nature does not display itself; the creative scientist must search for unity in hidden likenesses. We are dependent on the creative thinkers for the development of science.

Other attitudes that must be cultivated in the nurse researcher include the ability to be objective, the ability to stop and think, and the ability to define and express concepts. In addition, the nurse researcher needs to be able to live with "eternal uncertainty," generalize findings, and learn from mistakes. These qualities are in direct conflict with the traditional nurse role (Wald and Leonard, cited in Fox & Leeser, 1981).

The traditional nurse role has been one of dependency, not autonomy. Nurses have been socialized to act immediately, and task orientation has been a hallmark of the profession for years. Furthermore, nurses have been taught to live in fear of making mistakes, such as medication errors, and not to view their errors as productive failures. Nurses have been taught to operate in the all-or-none theory: thinking in absolutes rather than in the gray areas of possibility. The evolution of these research qualities in nurses is analogous to a metamorphosis. New patterns of action need to be developed by a large percentage of nurses before they have the mental flexibility to take on research responsibilities in their professional careers.

Rettig (1980) has identified four other characteristics that are as important to the success of the new nurse researcher as those listed above and are probably more important to the long-term survival of the nurse researcher. They are courage, discipline, patience, and humor.

Courage is necessary not only for obtaining approval to conduct research but also for facing problems that arise during the implementation phase of the study.

Discipline is required to write research proposals and to conduct research as well as to initiate any kind of research program in a service setting. Discipline is exercised when a flaw is found in a proposal design that has already been approved and ready for the implementation phase. Although the flaw itself may not jeopardize the research, the temptation to correct the flaw is great. Restraint must be exercised in order to maintain the proposal design as was originally submitted and approved for implementation.

While nursing research must not unduly disrupt patient care, it is apparent that patience is necessary when dealing with those doing the data collection. When the research study becomes a low priority in a service setting because of other unit crises, the researcher must be patient but flexible in pursuing research priorities. This latter example is a prevalent conflict for CNSs engaged in clinical research and will be addressed at a later point in the chapter.

The use of humor is a valuable method by which the nurse researcher can gain the cooperation of nursing staff and patients as well as an effective way to handle the stress and tension associated with research itself.

RESEARCH ACTIVITIES OF THE CNS

There are a variety of research activities that can be incorporated into the CNS role. Often it will not be possible to accomplish some of the higher level research activities until certain factors are in place that support nursing research within the service setting. It is wise for the CNS to begin from the most basic levels of research and work up the ladder of sophistication as the role of the CNS matures both from a personal perspective and from the perspective of the organization in which the CNS is employed.

The CNS and the Research Role

The CNS can be an ideal practitioner-scientist. By virtue of the CNS's graduate education, formal exposure to research methodology has occurred and a recognition of the value of nursing research has emerged as the CNS has prepared for specialty practice (Niessner, 1979).

Just as the literature has described various facets of the role of the CNS, Bowie (1980) has outlined eight roles of the nurse researcher: the researcher in the consumer, participative, supportive, technical, consultative, investigative, collaborative, and interpretive roles. These various research roles will be considered in greater detail in the next section of this chapter.

Bowie (1980) further states that the nurse researcher has responsibilities to the profession that include six distinct areas:

1. to be aware of gaps in scientific knowledge,
2. to establish priorities in accordance with nursing needs,
3. to ensure the integrity of research study designs,
4. to identify areas for further study,
5. to make research findings available to consumers, and
6. to follow up with further studies.

If one adheres to these responsibilities, a cyclical nature can develop. One research study often raises more questions than it answers!

Although many CNSs are reluctant to venture into the world of nursing research, once they enter, they are often held captive because of the many new questions that arise. The trick is to take that first step in becoming involved in nursing research. The cliche that "the perfect are the enemy of the good" is very applicable to nursing research. As Jacox (1974, p. 385) states, "If the researcher waits to start until she has a perfect design, she may never start. There has to be a careful balance between rigorous research and realistic expectations." This is particularly true for the CNS who is involved with nursing research as only one of the roles of the position.

The CNS need not conduct on-the-job research that is equivalent to a doctoral dissertation in order to fulfill the research-related aspects of her position. As was mentioned earlier in the chapter, research is the most sophisticated level of problem solving. This does not make the lower levels of problem solving (nursing process, POMR, and nursing audits) any less important. CNSs need to examine where they are in terms of research development within their role. While it is true that some CNSs conduct original clinical research, others may be promoting the spirit of inquiry in staff nurses to a greater extent by their very presence and questioning attitude than is typically apparent during the delivery of nursing care on a specific unit. The research process may also be apparent through various projects such as the development of patient classification systems or unit surveys that improve practice with more immediacy than does research. The success of CNSs in conducting research is dependent more on the establishment of a critical attitude than on the number of formal research proposals that list the CNS as the principal investigator.

Levels of Research Sophistication

Just as there are levels of sophistication in problem solving, so too are there levels of sophistication within the research process. In a broad sense, the CNS can either participate in nursing research or initiate research.

Stetler (1984) has identified four major levels of research: facilitating research by others, utilizing the research process in routine problem solving, utilizing research findings, and conducting research.

Facilitating research by other nurses includes activities such as deriving questions for study through the delivery of nursing care and involvement as data collectors for nurse researchers. Facilitating research can also be viewed as participating in research. This may require CNSs to complete surveys or questionnaires about their roles or to be a participant of research in some other form.

Utilization of the research process includes those activities already mentioned that are on the continuum of patient care evaluation. Facilitating and utilizing research correlate with the participative and supportive role of the nurse researcher.

Utilization of research findings is Stetler's (1984) third level of nursing research and corresponds with the interpretive and consumer role of the nurse researcher. This is the level in which research is applied in practice. By contrast, Hodgman (cited in Hamric & Spross, 1983) views the interpretation, evaluation, and communication of research findings to staff nurses as one of the most basic levels of research activity for the CNS. Actual testing and application of nursing research that is generated by others is seen as the second level of nursing research. For this reason, Hodgman describes these two activities as different levels of research utilization.

The application of research is viewed as an extremely important aspect of nursing research. Its importance is so great that a model to assist nurses in deciding if a research study should be applied in practice has been developed by Stetler and Marram (1976).

In the Stetler–Marram (p. 560) model for the utilization of research findings in practice, once a piece of research is critiqued and considered valid, four areas become factors in deciding whether to apply a research study in practice. These factors include substantiating evidence (existence of similar studies), the "fit" of the study (how similar the setting of the study is with the setting in which the research is to be applied), the feasibility (the availability of certain equipment, ethical risks, etc.), and the basis for practice (an indication of the effectiveness of current practice and its relationship to scientific rationale). If these critical factors are not met, the study should not be applied in the specific setting for which the model was used to evaluate applicability. If, however, the critical factors are satisfied, the nurse has the choice of cognitively applying the research findings so that the findings of the study become part of the theory base that is drawn upon in clinical practice or of directing application of the study through a more formal route. The nurse may opt to implement the change and evaluate the outcome, present the findings to administration or to peers for consideration, or institute a systematic evaluation of the designated practice within the new setting. As Stetler and Marram (1976) state, all cases of application involve testing the validity of the findings in the new setting and can therefore be considered "research in action." Applying research in the practice setting requires careful thought and deliberation.

The conduct of research is the last of Stetler's four levels of nursing research. It correlates with the technical, consultative, collaborative, and investigative roles of the nurse researcher. The conduct of research can be further divided into two levels: replication research and original research.

Replication research is the lower of the two levels of the conduct of research but is no less important than original research. In fact, Stetler (1983) believes that one of the major contributions that nurses in practice settings can make to the science of nursing is the conduct of replications. Stetler states (p. 208): "If knowledgeable nurses in multiple settings repeat scientific investigations and report their findings in the literature, then a sufficient body of knowledge may eventually exist to truly provide nursing with a scientific base for practice." Replication research may indeed be an option for the beginning researcher who wants the experience of conducting research but has neither the time nor the commitment to generate original research.

Original research consists of new studies that arise from questions to be answered from the nurse's personal experience with patient care. Original research also includes those studies in which the researcher may find a partial answer to a question in the literature but wishes to test another variable or hypothesis that may affect the outcome of the study.

Original research is the most sophisticated level of research and therefore requires the greatest skill and expertise on the part of the nurse researcher. In developing original research, the CNS follows the formal outline for proposals, which includes a problem statement, rationale for and significance of the study, review of what is already in the literature, a theoretical framework, specific hypotheses, questions, and purposes as well as details on the methodology to be used. The methodology includes the definition of terms used in the study in addition to information about the sample, population, instrumentation, design, procedure, and statistical analysis to be used. Details about these various components can be obtained from review of any number of research texts on the market.

CREATING AN ATMOSPHERE CONDUCIVE TO CLINICAL RESEARCH

Although the number of hospitals with nurse researchers and nursing research committees are growing, there are still many places where the concept of nurses doing research is quite foreign. If the CNS finds herself in a setting that has formalized its nursing research activities through committees and boards or has the luxury of having a nurse researcher on staff, the CNS by all means should utilize these resources to the maximum in order to facilitate the conduct of clinical nursing research within her role. Many CNSs, however, find that there is not an atmosphere of support readily available to them in research endeavors. It is for this reason that it is necessary to focus on the preliminary activities that must be addressed within the service setting before higher level nursing research can be a realistic expectation of the CNS.

Assessment of the Self

In institutions where there is no formal mechanism for the accomplishment of nursing research, the CNS is often looked to for direction in the establishment of such a program. Before a program can be initiated by the CNS, a close self-evaluation must occur. The basic qualities that are essential in any nurse researcher must also be apparent in the CNS. If the CNS is not open to new and different approaches to nursing care or does not have a belief and commitment to the development of nursing research, the implementation of research will not be successful.

Not only must the CNS have the attitudes and characteristics mentioned earlier in the chapter but the CNS must also have a certain degree of confidence with the role before research endeavors are undertaken. From the author's experience, it may take a minimum of 6–9 months in the unstructured role of the CNS to learn the position expectations and role requirements and to feel comfortable with the staff and the institutional policies and procedures. The conduct of original research is not an expectation that can be added to the CNS's job responsibilities during that first year of specialty practice. This does not mean that the research process cannot be utilized by the CNS in her first year of practice. In fact, the involvement of the CNS in the research process through other activities may very well serve the dual purpose of encouraging immediate changes that improve practice and building self-confidence in the CNS's research skills.

Readiness to be involved in nursing research is a personal decision. CNSs will all have different amounts of enthusiasm for research and therefore must evaluate their own commitment to this phase of their professional development. While self-evaluation of individuals involved in research is important, Stevenson (cited in Downs & Fleming, 1979) believes that there should be less emphasis on the individual in research and more of a focus on departmental acceptance of nursing research within the larger health care institutions.

Assessing Where Nursing Research "Fits" into the Organization

Eight organizational conditions have been identified by Egan, McElmurry, and Jameson (1981) that affect the ease with which nursing research will be accepted within a service setting. Among these are the availability of participants for studies, professional participants, market factors, organizational systems, economic factors, legal and/or statutory provisions, facilities and resources, and contributions to the research endeavors by local educational institutions. Before attempting to conduct practice-oriented research, it would be wise for the CNS to investigate each of these areas.

Access to human subjects for research is much more of a problem for researchers in academia than for most CNSs. However, the same guidelines that assure proper use of human subjects for a nurse in a faculty role will apply to the CNS as well. Any research involving the use of human subjects must be approved by institutional review boards designed specifically to safeguard the rights of patients.

Questions that will help to assess the level of subject participation that one could expect in research include the following: Have patients been asked to participate in research before? What was their response? Is the population that is being studied large enough in the particular setting to allow for a representative sample? What is the staff's background with nursing research? Would they be able to understand and participate in the study? Could nursing staff be utilized in data collection? Would there be an interest in doing so?

Market factors are defined by Egan et al. (1981) as the receptiveness of the nursing department (and other departments within the associated medical center) to nursing research and the demand for such a program. If other departments are in the dark as to the need for nursing research or do not view nursing as a distinct body of knowledge that is separate from the medical profession, it will indeed be difficult to make progress with the establishment and acceptance of a formalized program for nursing research within the institution.

Market factors can be assessed by the CNS with questions such as: How much time is allocated to patient surveys and utilization of the information gained from them? Are there multidisciplinary systematic studies presently being conducted within the medical center? Is research included in the mission statement of the hospital? If the CNS is practicing in a private hospital that does not have a strong mission toward research or an affiliation with a university, it will take much longer for nursing research to become recognized as an expectation of clinical practice.

The organizational system is closely related to market factors. Egan et al. (1981) states that the relation of hospital administration to a nursing department's systematic studies program is crucial. How do nursing and medicine approach quality assurance projects that affect the practices of both of their disciplines? Does the institution have a nursing department systematic studies program in the first place? If not, steps need to be taken to establish a strong nursing program in research before the relationship between the nursing studies program and its medical counterpart can be evaluated.

If the CNS is functioning in an institution where there is not a formal nursing research committee or program, the recent book authored by Stetler (1984) entitled *Nursing Research in a Service Setting* is recommended. The book is based on the nursing experience of Massachusetts General Hospital in setting up a nursing studies program of research. It includes many practical hints on how to initiate such a program and includes forms and exhibits that are invaluable to the nurse embarking on such a project.

Questions that assess the economic aspect of research readiness in the institution include those questions that investigate the current patterns for funding the programs and the personnel necessary to keep them functioning. In addition, the manner in which past research studies have been funded and the benefits and incentives that have been derived from the studies implemented are also important economic questions to consider before conducting nursing research in the service setting.

The first study often sets a precedent for future consideration of nursing research. Thus, it goes without saying that the first nursing study to go through a formal institutional review should be of high quality. Kerlinger (1977, p. 11) states, "Research that is not excellent has no place in science." It is difficult to make a second first impression. Along the same line of thought, it may be helpful for the CNS to select a topic that has wide interest among nurses in the institution rather than a study that would only impact on the practice of a few nurses who interact with a limited group of patients. The benefits of such research will be much greater and help to legitimize nursing research more quickly than a study that has an impact on fewer nurses and clients.

Another question that must be asked when evaluating an institution's research climate is whether or not an institutional review board (IRB) or its equivalent exists within the institution. More than likely, there will be a review board that will at least protect the rights of human subjects involved in research. It would behoove the CNS to meet with the chairperson of the board long before the time when a nursing proposal may be considered on the agenda. In settings where nurses have never done research, much education of both nurses and other individuals who have an interest in research (including those who are members of the IRB) will be necessary.

Facilities and resources are extremely important aspects of the institution that the CNS needs to become familiar with. Is there a medical library within the hospital that is easy to access? Is it staffed with a librarian who would be able to assist with literature searches, duplicating, and so on? Is there access to a health science library within a local university? Does the CNS have a library card that will allow utilization of the resources available? Where can the CNS find computer resources? Is there a research supervisor in the hospital Information Services Department? Is consultation with a statistician available through the hospital or a local university? If so, the CNS should get to know those people. Making personal contact and establishing rapport with key personnel will greatly enhance the opportunities surrounding all phases of the research process. Does the nursing department operate with personal computers? Can word-processing capabilities be extended to the CNS during proposal development? These are all factors that must be taken into consideration when first beginning to implement research in a service setting.

The final component in the model proposed by Egan et al. (1981) is the evaluation of the contributions to research endeavors by educational institutions. The local university can be a wealth of information for the beginning nurse researcher. Universities have historically provided the locus for philosophical and historical inquiries in all fields and professions. The social mission of higher institutions of learning has been threefold: teaching, service, and research (Schlotfeldt, 1977). The CNS practicing within a service setting does a disservice to herself and to the institution if she does not take the opportunity to link up with faculty from the local university.

Educational contributions to practice research include not only collaborative research between practitioners and faculty but also the contributions of student nurses within their clinical rotation. What clinical areas are important areas for research for the educational programs associated with the hospital? What are the student's preparation and goals in nursing research? Could students be utilized for data collection as a part of their exposure to nursing research? Could this be accomplished through an independent study for credit? The possibilities are endless.

Another ingredient that is crucial to the facilitation of a research atmosphere within an institution is the support of the nurse administrator. Someone in authority needs to set the example that nursing research is an important activity and one that the department as well as the profession sees as a legitimate use of time and energy. Without the support of the nurse administrator, nursing research by a CNS cannot become a reality.

In summary, nursing research is facilitated by certain characteristics within the service setting. Schlotfeldt (1977, p. 4) states, "The key predictor of nursing's eventual fulfillment of its potential as a socially significant, scientific, humanistic, learned profession is commitment to research, as it is expressed by individuals, by the corporate profession, and by institutions." The responsibility for creating the atmosphere rests not only with the CNS but also with the administrators and the institution itself.

TECHNIQUES FOR SUCCESSFUL RESEARCH IMPLEMENTATION

The process of implementing nursing research within a service setting is a challenge for most CNSs. It is a difficult task to initiate research because of the many obstacles that can interfere. Lack of administrative support and lack of knowledge about the research process, the nature of the traditional role of the nurse, problems inherent in the conduct of clinical research itself, and CNS role conflict can all impede the success of the CNS in incorporating the research component into the CNS role.

Overcoming Barriers to Clinical Nursing Research

Lack of institutional support is just one of a number of barriers to nursing research that the CNS may experience in trying to fulfill the research component of the role. Although the establishment of a climate for nursing research may be very slow, it is the first step in facilitating nursing research in a service setting. Nursing studies that are specific and short term and that lead to visible clinical feedback can be an excellent vehicle for initiating nursing research. Another avenue for establishing a positive research climate is the participation of faculty from neighboring universities in quality assurance projects. This may help raise awareness of the research process within the service setting as well as provide role models and resource persons for the CNS.

Administrative support from the nursing department is imperative in order for the CNS to successfully implement the research role. A monetary commitment by the nurse manager in the budget is probably the strongest statement of administrative support. However, even if funds are not allocated by the nursing department for nursing research, other supportive activities can be considered and implemented.

The establishment of a nursing research committee within the department greatly facilitates the introduction of nursing research in the practice setting. As chairperson of such a committee, the CNS can reach many staff nurses with the message that nursing research is a valued part of each nurse's professional practice. The goal of such a committee is usually to support, facilitate, encourage, and promote nursing research within the institution. While nurs-

ing research committees may serve as formal review boards for nursing proposals, the focus during the early stages of committee development should
be on the facilitation of research in general rather than on specific projects
(Padilla, 1979).

Before the goals of a nursing research committee can be operationalized,
the staff nurses must be familiar with the research process. Lack of understanding of the research process is yet another barrier that the CNS must
address when directing a research program or committee.

Ways that a nursing research committee (or a CNS individually) can help
to raise the level of awareness of research within the staff nurse population
include formal inservices about the research process and clinical seminars in
which the staff are exposed to nursing research through guest speakers who
discuss the research they have conducted or some other aspect of the research
process. Since it is so very difficult for staff nurses to get away from the unit,
a brown bag luncheon may be an effective way to critique published nursing
research and provide inservice at the same time. By choosing research that
is of interest to the participants, lively discussion can be evoked that may
subsequently lead to application of the research in practice (if appropriate)
or generate ideas for further study.

Since many states as well as institutions have continuing education requirements for their employees, it would be wise to work with the inservice
education department in order to secure continuing education credits for attending research-based inservices. Other ideas include awarding inservice
credit for staff nurses who wish to participate in actual data collection for a
clinical study or for assisting the CNS with a research study by doing a literature review.

The traditional role of the nurse has been mentioned previously as being
a barrier to the effective implementation of research in the service setting. A
resocialization of nurses needs to occur so that the research role becomes an
unquestioned aspect of patient care. Staff nurses have often voiced the opinion that research is a responsibility that lies outside of nursing service.

CNSs who actually conduct nursing research may be harassed by staff
nurses because of the CNS's lack of visibility on the unit and access to her
during the time of proposal development. Girouard (cited in Hamric &
Spross, 1983) believes that involving staff in the research effort and focusing
on research that investigates clinical problems shared by others will facilitate
the inclusion of the research role within the staff nurse's responsibilities and

the staff's acceptance of the CNS's desire to conduct clinical research. Jacox (1974, p. 382) states:

> If we are to have knowledge that is useful for practice, then a majority of the persons who develop that knowledge must be so familiar with the clinical setting that they are able to identify truly significant problems for study. Nursing can never develop a scientific basis for its practice until the practitioners themselves — not just the "career" researchers — have a great deal more involvement in the research.

In addition to the lack of institutional support, lack of understanding of the research process by staff nurses, and the problems identified with the traditional role of the nurse, Padilla (1979) also identifies lack of patient support as a barrier that can deter clinical nursing research from occurring in the practice setting. She suggests that nurse researchers exercise great care in drafting patient consent forms and explaining studies to patients so that they will be more likely to participate in the investigations.

Problems Inherent in Clinical Nursing Research

The conduct of clinical research has a few inherent problems of its own even if the climate in the institution is very conducive to research. Jacox (1974) indentifies three areas that warrant careful consideration before beginning clinical research: procuring the sample, measuring clinical phenomena, and controlling extraneous variables.

Obtaining representative groups for the sample is often problematic for the clinical researcher. It is important for the researcher to know what kind of population is essential for the study being conducted and the accessibility of the group. In some studies, an option may be to have the subject serve as his own controlled match if achieving a matched sample is desirable but not possible.

The measurement of clinical phenomena is difficult because no matter to what extent we have gone in order to assure precise measurement, we are dealing with human nature. Often we are not measuring what we think we are measuring. In addition, "people are reluctant to say that they are dissatisfied with the care they are receiving while they are receiving it," (Nehring and Geach cited in Jacox, 1974, p. 384).

The practice setting is often plagued by last-minute changes that can affect a research study being conducted on a nursing unit. Fluctuations in patient acuity and staffing patterns are examples of occurrences that may adversely impact the conduct of research.

While these areas of problems in clinical research require attention by the CNS, the same problems are experienced by other health professionals dealing with research in the practice setting. These problems cannot be used as excuses for not attempting clinical research.

Dealing with Role Conflict

Role conflict is a phenomenon that occurs frequently with CNSs because of the lack of clarity regarding the role itself. With research being only one small part of the role, it is no wonder that the CNS feels pulled in various directions. The CNS is often expected to be all things to all people. Because the research role can require much time before results are seen, the CNS may opt to invest time in another area of practice that will reap benefits sooner. This is particularly true of the CNS who is just beginning clinical specialty practice.

Wooldrige, Leonard, and Skipper (1978) have identified some aspects of the research role that may set the CNS up for conflict. Because the CNS is a relatively young role within the profession, many CNSs are themselves very young. Often the young nurse or the nurse with less experience is also seen as being less knowledgeable and therefore is more prone to having research criticized or rejected. CNSs who conduct research in nursing are also likely to demonstrate through their studies that, for example, the current method of staffing is not as effective as another method. Nurses doing nursing research may very well fail to clearly differentiate between medical and nursing care. In both instances, the research could result in criticism of the work of others (administrators or physicians) who have a higher status in the organization. To say the least, this situation would be very awkward for the CNS.

All CNSs are keenly aware of the many demands placed on their time. On some days, dealing with the pressures that increasingly exist on the unit level may be all that the CNS can handle. Assuring that the daily demands for patient care are met is certainly a priority for the hospital and would take precedence over the conduct of clinical research. Each CNS needs to determine when the timing is right to concentrate efforts on research. It is much easier to focus on one aspect of the CNS role for a certain time period. During that time, research (for example) may be the emphasis of practice but not to the exclusion of the other roles of clinician, educator, consultant, and manager.

Although it is difficult to separate these various roles, when dealing with nursing research, it is quite beneficial to devote a block of time to the research process. Klein and Johnston (1979) recommended that the health care worker who conducts research take special care to clearly identify the exact role played by the researcher during the conduct of studies. The CNS who is conducting a study on a postoperative unit, for example, can very easily get called to patient rooms to assess postoperative bleeding or to assist patients to manage pain. Some CNSs wear a different color or length of lab coat when collecting data. By being straightforward with the staff and letting them know exactly why the CNS is on the unit, the CNS can eliminate or at least minimize negative feelings among the staff.

The conduct of nursing research is important, and the CNS has a responsibility to foster a climate within the institution so that nursing research can occur. Niesser (1979, p. 25) states:

> The CNS must not allow herself to become so involved in the daily pressures and demands of the organization that she delegates scientific inquiry to a low, almost negligible priority. Nursing will never develop a truly scientific basis for its practice until the practitioners themselves accept increasing involvement in the research process.

IDENTIFYING SUPPORT GROUPS FOR RESEARCH

Because many institutions do not have an abundance of CNSs, it is very easy for the CNS to feel isolated. A key aspect of surviving both the CNS role and the research role lies in the establishment of peer support and professional networks. Just as research activities are classified in levels, so too are the support groups that exist for nursing research. There are formalized groups that exist on national, state, and local levels. In addition, informal groups may also exist within various communities. The CNS who is beginning to conduct nursing research may gain the most emotional support from the local level, where an exchange can occur among colleagues who have experienced the same barriers to research that are problematic for the CNS.

Peer support is extremely helpful to the CNS who needs to know that others have been through the same process and have indeed been able to implement research within the same community where the CNS practices.

Local Nursing Research Support Groups

The best place for the CNS to find support is among those closest to her: peers in the work place. The nursing research committee of the nursing department serves a very ego-strengthening purpose. It is easy to become overwhelmed with details when first beginning research, and the nursing research committee members can help to keep things in perspective and to encourage one another in research efforts.

It is important, however, that the chairperson of such a committee chooses the members carefully. When possible, it is preferable to have at least one member (other than the CNS) who is prepared at the master's level. Encouraging participation from staff nurses who are critical thinkers, however, is just as important and should not be overlooked.

Nursing research committees should have a staff nurse membership component. Davis (1981, pp. 25–26) states:

> The work involved in research is not well known or understood. Clinical nurses have to discover what a research work rhythm is, that is, how much research work is reasonable to expect from oneself within a specific period of time. Through their actual involvement in research, they experience the differences between the clinical and research work rhythms.

Because the nature of research requires long periods of time to see the results of efforts, the core group of members on the committee need to stay fairly consistent over a number of years. The nursing research committee is not a departmental committee that should change membership on a yearly basis. The supportive nature of such a committee would diminish if the group consistently needed to deal with updating new members on what had taken place within the committee.

It has already been mentioned that the participation of faculty in clinical research is beneficial. Having a faculty member serve as an advisory member on a nursing research committee is a valuable component to the success of such a committee and should not be downplayed.

Collaborative research between faculty and practitioners should be encouraged. The CNS may be able to invite a faculty person to be coinvestigator. The coinvestigator may help to obtain access to library facilities. Faculty can also be invaluable during the data analysis phase of research. Choosing a faculty member who has earned a doctoral degree is helpful to assure expertise in the use of statistical analysis. The actual collection of data from patients, however, may be easier for the CNS to facilitate and direct than for the faculty person since the CNS has greater access to patients in the service setting. The trade-offs between the CNS and the faculty person can be negotiated with minimal difficulty, and the end result can be excellent clinical nursing studies.

The local district nurses association is the next place the CNS can seek peer support for research efforts. Most districts have special-interest groups in existence. Even if there is not a specific nursing research group, there may be a CNS group that could lend support to other CNSs in research endeavors. If there is not a research interest group in your local area, why not begin one? Identifying nurses in the community who are doing research is the first step in establishing a networking and support group.

Regional and State Support Groups

The next level of support groups for research exists on the state and regional level. As is the case with district nurse associations, there are a number of state nurse associations that have state councils that belong to the ANA Council of Nurse Researchers which was formed in the early 1970s with the intent of providing a reference group and a forum where nurse researchers could meet and collaborate around common interests (Stevenson, cited in Downs & Fleming, 1979). The state councils work toward the same purpose as the district research groups but focus on the convening of statewide seminars and other research activities that will help to achieve the overall goals of the council. Information about state councils of nurse researchers can be obtained from state nurse associations.

Regional organizations also exist that can help to support and encourage nursing research. These groups include the Western Interstate Commission of Higher Education in Nursing (WICHEN), the Southern Regional Education Board (SREB), and the Committee on Institutional Cooperation (CIC). WICHEN is a powerful promoter of nursing research in the following 13 states: Alaska, Arizona, California, Colorado, Hawaii, Idaho, Montana, Nevada, New Mexico, Oregon, Utah, Washington, and Wyoming. The 14 states serviced by the SREB are Alabama, Arkansas, Florida, Georgia, Kentucky, Louisiana, Maryland, Mississippi, North Carolina, South Carolina, Tennessee, Texas, Virginia, and West Virginia. Lastly, the CIC is a consortium in the midwest composed of the big-ten universities: Illinois, Indiana, Iowa, Michigan, Michigan State, Minnesota, Northwestern, Ohio State, Purdue, and Wisconsin (Stevenson, cited in Downs & Fleming, 1979). All of these regional support groups can be valuable to the CNS who would like to meet and benefit from the experiences of other more seasoned researchers.

National Support Groups for Nursing Research

There are a variety of national organizations that can be considered support groups for nurses engaged in nursing research. The ANA Council of Nurse Researchers provides an atmosphere for sharing nursing research that is in progress in addition to the reference group function. The ANA Council of Nurse Researchers has a variety of research-related activities for the membership, including the publication of a research newsletter.

Other national groups that have expressed a commitment to nursing research include the National League for Nursing (NLN), the American Nurse's Foundation (ANF), Sigma Theta Tau, and the American Association of Critical Care Nurses (AACN). NLN was instrumental in the establishment of early funding for projects in nursing research. Both the ANF and Sigma Theta Tau award small grants to nurses conducting research. The ultimate goal of all of these groups is to facilitate and encourage the development of nursing research within our country.

The CNS has a multitude of places to turn in search of support for scholarly research endeavors. While these support groups were presented in this chapter in a very abbreviated form, the reader is encouraged to further investigate how these groups may be of significant assistance to the CNS in enactment of the research role.

COMMITMENT TO RESEARCH

The responsibility of the CNS to the pursuit of new nursing knowledge cannot be taken lightly. Nor should the CNS be satisfied with the mere conduct of research. Unless there is an active exchange between those generating new knowledge and those using the knowledge, the advancement of the science of nursing will never occur (Bloch, 1980).

It is extremely important that the CNS shares research findings with others through publications and/or research presentations. Staff who have participated in research should be extended the results of the study prior to dissemination of the findings to other sources (Chance & Hinshaw, 1980). This is a courtesy to the staff and helps them to accept nursing research. Similarly, health care administrators need to be kept appraised of the progress and findings of studies. Wooldridge et al. (1978, p. 181) state:

> Although one of the goals of the researchers may be to make their findings known to as many interested professionals as possible, home base can be covered. Researchers have an obligation to make their findings known to any sponsoring or funding agency and the officials of the institution in which the research took place before the general public.

There are a number of nursing journals interested in publishing nursing research. For specific publication requirements of individual journals, see Martinson (1981).

The motivation necessary to conduct nursing research is a highly individual matter. For some, motivation comes from outside of themselves. External motivating factors include promotion and salary increases. For others, motivation is an internal force. Research is done because there is a burning desire from within to solve a question, to approach a problem from a different perspective, or to attempt something that has never been done before. Regardless of the motivating forces for research, the degree of motivation and commitment by CNSs to research will differ. Some CNSs who value research may not have the qualities needed to successfully conduct original research. Others with the needed qualities may not value this aspect of professional nursing.

Regardless of the recommendation by the nursing profession that CNSs should conduct nursing research, the decision to participate in a specific level of research is ultimately an individual one on the part of the CNS. The CNS must evaluate where research fits within personal and professional goals. Is research something that is personally valued? Will research provide the CNS with professional growth? What are the rewards of conducting research? Are they sufficient to encourage the CNS to undertake a research study? The CNS's commitment to nursing research is the key ingredient to success in the research role.

Clinical practice is what the profession of nursing is all about, and CNSs are in a position to have a profound impact on clinical nursing practice. Diers (1979, p. 4) states:

No amount of research can ever destroy the personal satisfaction that comes from giving excellent patient care, nor can any amount of research ever predict or prescribe all the nursing care for an individual patient. But research can provide information on which to base decisions about patient care. As we learn more about what in nursing brings about the desired effects for patients, the patient care gets better and better, and that's the whole purpose for nursing research.

The CNS can be both a practitioner and a scholar. As more CNSs include research activities into their positions, the title could very well change. The "clinical nurse scientist" (a new "CNS") may soon be born.

BIBLIOGRAPHY

ANA (1980, December). *Nursing—A social policy statement*. Code # NP-63, 35M. New York: American Nurses Association

Bloch, D. (1980). Interrelated issues in evaluation and evaluation research. *Nursing Research*, **29**(2), 69–73.

Bowie, R. B. (1980). The nurse researcher's roles and responsibilities. *AORN Journal*, **31**(4), 609–611.

Brown, M. (1981). Research in the development of nursing theory: The importance of a theoretical framework in nursing research. In Fox, D. J., & Leeser, I. (Eds.), *Readings on the research process in nursing*. New York: Appleton-Century-Crofts.

Bush, C. T. (1985). *Nursing research*. Reston, VA: Reston.

Chance, H. C., & Hinshaw, A. S. (1980). Strategies for initiating a research program. *Journal of Nursing Administration*, **10**(3), 32–39.

Cormack, D. F. (Ed.). (1984). *The research process in nursing*. London: Blackwell.

Davis, M. Z. (1981). Promoting nursing research in the clinical setting. *Journal of Nursing Administration*, **11**(3), 22–27.

Diers, D. (1979). *Research in nursing practice*. New York: Lippincott.

Downs, F., & Fleming, J. (1979). *Issues in nursing research*. New York: Appleton-Century-Crofts.

Egan, E. C., McElmurry, B. J., & Jameson, H. M. (1981). Practice-based research: Assessing your department's readiness. *Journal of Nursing Administration*, **11**(10), 26–36.

Folta, J. R. (1975). Conference on the nature of science and nursing: Perspectives of an applied scientist. In Gortner, S. R., 1975, Research for a practice profession. *Nursing Research*, **24**(3), 193–197.

Fox, D. J., & Leeser, I. (1981). *Readings on the research process in nursing*. New York: Appleton-Century-Crofts.

Girouard, S. (1983). Implementing the research role. In Hamric, A. B., & Spross, J. (Eds.), *The clinical nurse specialist in theory and practice* (pp. 83–89). New York: Grune & Stratton.

Gortner, S. R. (1975). Research for a practice profession. *Nursing Research*, **24**(3), 193–197.

Gortner, S. R. (1979). Trends and historical perspective. In Downs, F., & Fleming, J. (Eds.), *Issues in nursing research* (pp. 1–23). New York: Appleton-Century-Crofts.

Hamric, A. B., & Spross, J. (Eds.). (1983). *The clinical nurse specialist in theory and practice*. New York: Grune & Stratton.

Henderson, V. A. (1956). Research in nursing practice—when? (Editorial). *Nursing Research*, **4**(3), 99.

Hinshaw, A. S., Chance, H. C., & Atwood, J. (1981). Research in practice: A process of collaboration and negotiation. *Journal of Nursing Administration*, **11**(2), 33–36.

Hodgman, E. C. (1983). The CNS as researcher. In Hamric, A. B. & Spross, J. (Eds.), *The clinical nurse specialist in theory and practice* (pp. 73–82). New York: Grune & Stratton.

Jacox, A. (1974). Nursing research and the clinician. *Nursing Outlook*, **22**(6), 382–385.

Jacox, A., & Prescott, P. (1978, November). Determining a study's relevance for clinical practice. *American Journal of Nursing*, **78**(11), 1882–1889.

Johnson, D. E. (1981). The nature of a science of nursing. In Fox, D. J., & Leeser, I. (Eds.), *Readings on the research process in nursing* (pp. 6–12). New York: Appleton-Century-Crofts.

Kerlinger, F. N. (1977, September). The influence of research on education practice. *Educational Researcher*, **6**, 5–12.

Klein, N., & Johnston, M. (1979). Insider-out: The health care worker as researcher. *Nursing Research*, **28**(5), 312–314.

Leininger, M. M. (Ed.). (1985). *Qualitative research methods in nursing*. New York: Grune & Stratton.

Marriner, A. (1979, December). The research process in quality assurance. *American Journal of Nursing*, **79**(12), 2158–2161.

Martinson, I. M. (Ed.). (1981). *Guide to publishing opportunities for nurses*. Minnesota: University of Minnesota School of Nursing.

Nehring, V., & Geach, B. (1973, May). Patients' evaluation of their care: Why they don't complain. *Nursing Outlook*, **21**, 317–321.

Newman, M. A. (1982). What differentiates clinical research? *Image*, **14**(3), 86–88.

Niessner, P. (1979). The clinical specialist's contribution to quality nursing care. *Nursing Leadership*, **2**, 21–30.

Notter, L. E. (1968, November–December). The nature of science and nursing (Editorial). *Nursing Research*, **17**, 483.

Padilla, G. (1979). Incorporating research in a service setting. *Journal of Nursing Administration*, **9**(1), 44–49.

Polit, D., & Hungler, B. (1985). *Nursing research principles and methods* (3rd ed.). Philadelphia: Lippincott.

Rettig, F. M. (1980). Ideal attitudes of a nurse researcher. *AORN Journal*, **32**(1), 62–64.

Schlotfeldt, R. (1977). Nursing research: Reflection of values. *Nursing Research*, **26**(1), 4–9.

Stetler, C. B. (1983, May/June). Nurses and research: Responsibility and involvement. *National Intravenous Therapy Association*, **6**, 207–212.

Stetler, C. B. (1984). *Nursing research in a service setting*. Reston, VA: Reston.

Stetler, C. B., & Marram, G. (1976). Evaluating research findings for applicability in practice. Nursing Outlook, **24**(9), 559–563.

Stevenson, J. S. (1979). Support for an emerging social institution. In Downs, F., & Fleming, J. (Eds.), *Issues in nursing research* (pp. 39–66). New York: Appleton-Century-Crofts.

Trussell, P., Brandt, A., & Knapp, S. (1981). *Using nursing research: Discovery, analysis, and interpretation*. Rockville, MD: Aspen Systems.

Wald, F. S., & Leonard, R. C. (1964). Towards development of a nursing practice theory. In Fox, D. J., & Leeser, I. (Eds.), *Readings on the research process in nursing* (pp. 17–23). New York: Appleton-Century-Crofts.

Wooldrige, P. J., Leonard, R. C., & Skipper, J. K. (1978). *Methods of clinical experimentation to improve patient care*. St. Louis: Mosby.

CASE STUDY: CNS AS RESEARCHER
Christy A. Price, M.S.N., R.N., C.C.R.N.

Getting started on a research project can appear like an insurmountable task. However, if one proceeds with appropriate guidance and in an organized fashion, it can develop into a very satisfying experience. Neophyte nursing researchers generally easily fulfill the first requirement of a research study. From their clinical experience and nursing career they have identified some aspect of professional nursing, patient care, or administrative conflict that would benefit from a critical examination.

Prior to becoming formally involved in research, I had been concerned about and questioned certain verbal and nonverbal behaviors that I frequently witnessed in the pediatric patients I cared for who had end-stage renal disease (ESRD) and required chronic hemodialysis. My colleagues who had been interacting with this patient population for several more years than I would explain these behaviors as unfortunate realities related to their disease and necessary treatment. These patients seemed overly immature and developmentally delayed when compared to their peers. This situation was disturbing and heavily influenced by nurse–patient relationships. I recognized a need to change the existing status quo. Therefore, I took on the challenge of hopefully documenting my clinical assumptions through a formal research study.

FORMULATING A ROUGH DRAFT

Having a sincere interest and dedication to nephrology nursing, I commenced the research process by writing a first, or rough, draft to present to the supervising professionals whom I had assessed as having the expertise for offering guidance with this project. The initial manuscript consisted of a brief outline describing the patient population, stating the hypotheses, and planning the methodology. All of the sections were refined as the study progressed. New researchers tend to be very much in need of having realistic limits and direction established by those with more experience. That is to say, my first drafts were much too verbose. A good author is accurate and stimulating but concise. It was difficult to "cut" material that I considered essential at the time.

Also included in this outline was a personal expression of why this study needed to be completed. A review of the literature along with my clinical assessments clearly demonstrated the area could benefit from further study. I had specific purposes in mind that I could share. I was able to generate a number of questions that could be answered by the research. My intentions were to improve the nursing care of ESRD patients through investigation of their developmental and vocational maturity and to attempt to establish some relationships between age of onset of kidney failure, number of years on hemodialysis, and an individual's developmental progression. A problem statement with all terms defined was included to assist all health care professionals in gaining an appreciation for the dynamics of the study. Finally, a review of the literature was presented that proved to become more extensive as the planned study solidified in its intent and organization.

The process of reviewing the literature definitely was a good experience, although it involved more than I had anticipated. I was primarily interested in the chronic renal failure literature, but in order to answer the research question, I was also led to other areas, including: chronic illness, vocational careers, developmental maturity, and psychosocial rehabilitation. This was necessary to make certain I was presenting a truly comprehensive search. At times reading nonnursing articles required extra cups of coffee and a stronger dose of determination.

SELECTING A STUDY POPULATION

Originally I had decided on a patient population of all hemodialysis patients 18 years old or younger in the local community. I had made a few informal contacts to gain a perspective on the number of subjects this would provide. Since I was involved in nephrology, although not pediatric dialysis at the time, I did not anticipate a major difficulty in contacting this patient population; however, I soon realized that the number of patients under 18 years of age was very limited. Additionally, I became more aware of the work involved, especially obtaining informed consent when the sample contains minors. After reevaluating the available population, new parameters were set at 10–24 years of age. This then meant that approximately half the subjects could provide informed consent without a parent being involved.

At the suggestion of my supervising committee, a next step was to evaluate using a control group of essentially healthy normal chronologically age-matched peers. This seemed very appropriate since my goal was to demonstrate developmental delay, or arrest. Finding a control group actually was not as difficult as I had expected; however, the time involved in the data collection phase was lengthy. Since the local medical center had a College of Dentistry that provided a pediatric training program, there was a number of 10–24-year-old individuals available who could be invited to serve as control group subjects.

Finally, it was also deemed of interest to compare the patients with chronic renal failure to others who had a chronic disease entity. Diabetes mellitus was chosen because of its juvenile onset classification. Also, there was available in the community a supportive pediatrician who specialized in chronic medical diseases.

Locating a study population can be time consuming. Generally, a researcher will know of her primary group, but recruiting comparison groups and control subjects requires thorough investigation of available community resources. Hospital contacts, other professionals, and the telephone directory were all utilized. Finding the population is the first step. From there I had to communicate by mail and engage in personal interviews with several administrators, physicians, and nurses to gain permission to approach their patients for participation in the study. Consent forms and cover letters had to be designed for each group.

For a researcher, much of this phase seems like unending paperwork. Historically, nurses have not gained the expertise in paper shuffling so this task often becomes an unwelcomed burden. I persisted in the preparing, collating, and processing of all the necessary forms.

I also realized that my past experience in public speaking and forensic debating was paying off nicely. My communication and interview skills were intact. However, I must admit that after I convinced everyone of the merits of my study, I started doubting myself. I would have to separate from the topic for a few days to regain a proper perspective in my research and life in general. This is not to say I was discouraged; rather I was encouraged. Every positive response brought a sense of accomplishment, another hill conquered on my way over the mountain.

STATING THE HYPOTHESES, ASSUMPTIONS, AND LIMITATIONS

From my professional journal reading and nursing care of pediatric patients with ESRD, I had formulated several hypotheses regarding the attitudes and behaviors of these patients. In order to remain as objective as possible, I decided on Erik Erikson's theory of life stages and progression through those stages as a conceptual framework and guide for development of my hypotheses. I formulated six hypotheses for the study based on the three study populations and the selected areas of psychosocial development and vocational maturity. The plan was to demonstrate developmental and vocational immaturity in the ESRD subjects when compared with either the diabetic subjects or essentially healthy peers. There was an intent also to demonstrate a greater immaturity the younger the patient was at the onset of his chronic renal failure and the longer time he had been on hemodialysis.

In the research design, it is essential that attention be given to the selection of appropriate tools that will provide the data for analysis. The Inventory of Psychosocial Development (IPD) measures the indices of Erikson's eight stages of life. Namely, trust versus mistrust, autonomy versus shame, initiative versus guilt, industry versus inferiority, identity versus role diffusion, and intimacy versus isolation were the six stages of developmental tasks utilized for this research. The IPD is a seven-point Likert-type self-rating scale. This instrument was first presented by Wessman and Ricks (1966) and then adopted by Constantinople (1970) and Evans (1979). Sixty statements were appropriate for the study population.

A second questionnaire, the Career Maturity Inventory (CMI) was selected after review of the literature to evaluate vocational maturity. The CMI was constructed by Crites (1965, 1971) to measure the indices identified by Super and co-worker's classic Career Pattern Study (1960, 1963). It is a 50-item questionnaire with a true–false format.

Two limitations of the study concerned the questionnaires. The IPD had never been tested on a similar sample population and lacked normative data. The CMI had available data only from grades 6 through 12, although it had been shown to be applicable through the senior year of college.

To locate these questionnaires, I had to utilize all available resources: my committee, peers in psychology, and social workers. They were able to offer suggestions for reference materials from which I could select tools. With their suggestions in hand, I cruised the library, which by this time had become my first home. I literally ploughed through reference materials too numerous to count. I used to chuckle when the library staff would greet me with, "We saved you a chair tonight." Even though they were seemingly questioning my sanity, I knew I would achieve my goal. I was beginning to feel like, and identify with, all researchers.

These two questionnaires and a demographic information sheet became my data collection tools. I wrote the authors of these instruments to obtain permission for their use in my study. I must admit it was an exciting moment when I received letters of support from those authors. Their letters remain in my file of significant memoirs.

A few assumptions were made, but two directly related to the theoretical frameworks of Erikson and Super. One had to assume that an individual normally develops according to the stages, or patterns outlined by these theorists. There is substantial work that supports the likelihood of this occurring if there are no prolonged interferences in an individual's formative years (Roazen, 1976).

METHODOLOGY FOR DATA COLLECTION

Having formalized the research, I proceeded to obtain written permission from all pertinent people. I then presented the research protocol to the Internal Review Board of the medical center. With the need, informed consents, and benefits of the study documented, permission was granted to start the process of data collection.

However, the IRB approval was not achieved without a few sleepless nights, skipped meals, and nervous moments. As I sat outside the conference room, I formulated plans on how I would personally persecute each member of the board if they dared to say no. I had conceived this "baby," and it had every right to grow to its full potential. The IRB vote of support was unanimous. They felt my proposal was well organized, complete in preparation, and potentially a contribution to society. Needless to say, I celebrated that night.

An exploratory, descriptive survey approach was chosen to study the selected areas of psychosocial development and maturity as identified by the IPD and CMI. With these questionnaires, a demographic sheet, and cover letter as my study packet, I began setting appointments to meet with the ESRD and diabetic patients in their respective clinic setting. Meetings were always arranged at the convenience of the patients or their parents, and the times ranged from 0700 to 2300 Monday through Saturday. I would meet with these individuals at the clinic, and after introductions were completed, I would spend 10–15 minutes explaining the nature of the study, my goals and anticipated benefits to the study populations. If the patient and/or a parent agreed to participate, and after their questions were answered, I would provide a study packet along with a stamped self-addressed envelope and request that the materials be returned in 3–4 days. Suggesting a time limit often enhances a prompt response and thereby a greater percentage of participation.

In this manner, I recruited 20 renal subjects with a data-producing sample of 14 subjects, or 70% of those invited. In the diabetic population, I recruited 13 subjects, and as with the renal patients, all indicated a willingness to participate. Of the 13 who agreed to participate, 8 (62%) of those contracted returned the questionnaires. These selected sample groups were limited by my time restraints and by utilizing one geographical area.

Finally, the control group was contacted in a similar fashion around their scheduled clinical appointments at the dental school. Fifty subjects were invited to participate, and all but one expressed a willingness to participate. Of the 49 who were provided packets 28 (57%) returned the questionnaires.

In summary, a total of 83 subjects were invited to participate in the study. From all three sample populations, a total of 50 questionnaires became data-producing samples for further analysis. The time involvement of the investigator can only be approximated at several hundred hours over a 4-month period. The expense involved included purchasing questionnaires, xeroxing cover letters and demographic sheets, and purchasing supplies such as envelopes and stamps.

I was about 8 months into my research, and the previous 4 months had actually been quite enjoyable. First, I was back with patients involved in a different approach to nursing care. Second, as the responses filled my mailbox and data collection took on a presentable form, I was getting something in return for my energy expenditure. Every questionnaire became an acknowledgement of my efforts.

DATA ANALYSIS BY STATISTICAL PROCEDURES

As the questionnaires were returned, I began tabulating the data. I designed flow sheets that would facilitate the work of data processing and statistical analysis by a computer programmer. There were a few communication and technical problems, which probably occur whenever a health care professional and a statistician discuss a research study.

There were several inaccurate runs of the data due mostly to inaccurate statistical help. Then there were interruptions because of staff summer vacations. Becoming very discouraged, I agreed to meet with another statistician, whose apologies for my inconveniences helped rekindle the spirit. The final data analysis was completed in an acceptable format.

Descriptive statistics were used to describe the sample and subsamples. Correlations revealed the nature and magnitude of the relationship between selected characteristics of the subjects and their psychosocial maturity as measured by the IPD. Pearson product–moment correlation coefficients between age in years and psychosocial development scores (which reached statistical significance) were illustrated in graphic form.

For this study one-way analysis of variance (ANOVA) was used to explore any differences among the three study samples on those subcategories of the IPD that fit the assumptions of parametric testing, that is, normal distribution curve and homogeneity of variance. Based on Erikson's developmental tasks for life stages, the variables of trust, mistrust, autonomy, shame, guilt, industry, inferiority, identity, and role diffusion were tested in this manner.

The three remaining variables of initiative, intimacy, and isolation could not be analyzed with parametric tests because the skewness of the distribution and kurtosis of the curve demonstrated a nonnormal distribution for the sample data. Likewise, the testing of vocational maturity, as measured by the CMI, required a nonparametric statistical procedure. For these variables, the statistical tests, Kruskal-Wallis with follow-up Mann-Whitney U, were performed.

This section may sound as if I have a real grasp for statistical analysis. Let me assure all readers that I spent many, many hours by candlelight trying to interpret the various meanings and approaches for discussion of research findings. My forte is not statistical computation and analysis, but nursing. However, a good researcher must be willing and able to discuss study results in a formal, objective style where all professionals can find common ground for understanding the project.

DISCUSSION OF THE FINDINGS

Presenting and discussing the findings after months of dedicated, diligent work are the highlights for a researcher. It is the time to shine for your accomplishment in perseverance toward a goal. An oral presentation allows the researcher the liberty of comfortably and sociably enlightening her peers. The feedback is immediate and, in my case, extremely positive for having completed an original research project in a very underinvestigated area of patient care. Also, the researcher gains the recognition of her colleagues and provides informative expertise for a select professional community by publishing the findings of a formal study. Both statistical and serendipitous findings for this study have been published (Price, 1982, 1984).

The final analysis and sharing of any research is testing the hypotheses. For my study, I was able to provide statistical confirmation for four of the six hypotheses.

In summary, the patients with ESRD on hemodialysis demonstrated less developmental maturity in the areas of guilt, role diffusion, and intimacy. When renal subjects were compared with essentially healthy peers, their scores on the vocational maturity scale represented greater immaturity, and the comparison was statistically significant. There were no statistically significant differences between the diabetics and the control group on the vocational maturity scale. Finally, the diabetic group did demonstrate greater developmental maturity than the renal group in the variables of guilt, role diffusion, intimacy and vocational maturity.

An additional serendipitous finding of this study was that the author found research not only worthwhile but also extremely satisfying. The research role of the clinical specialist provides a unique opportunity for self-expression and contribution to professional nursing.

CONCLUSION

The findings of this study must be viewed with caution in consideration of the small sample size. The differences that did surface offer some support for the researcher's clinical observations, assumptions, and experiences. All reported findings definitely contribute to nephrology nursing's understanding of the pediatric hemodialysis patient. While the sample size limited the number of statistically significant findings, the empirical data and coincidental discoveries strongly indicate that future investigation should address larger samples from different geographical localities to gain a universal picture. The end result would be enhanced nurse–patient relationships with an increased appreciation for the psychosocial and developmental problems of the patient population.

BIBLIOGRAPHY

Crites, J. (1965). Measurement of vocational maturity in adolescence. *Psychology Mongoraphs*, **79**(2), 1–36.

Crites, J. (1971). *The maturity of vocational attitudes in adolescence*. Washington, DC: American Personnel and Guidance Association.

Constantinople, A. (1970). An Eriksonian measure of personality development on college students. *Developmental Psychology*, **2**(3), 447.

Evans, A. (1979). An Eriksonian measure of personality development in child-abusing mothers. *Psychology Report*, **44**, 963–966.

Jordaan, J., & Heyde, M. (1960). *Vocational maturity during the high school years*. New York: Teachers College.

Price, C. (1982). Developmental maturity of adolescent and young adult patients on chronic hemodialysis: A comparative study. *AANNT Journal*, **9**(6), 17–20

Price, C. (1984). Parental behaviors: The effect on young patients with End Stage Renal Disease. *Journal of Nephrology Nursing*, **1**(1), 50–53.

Roazen, P. (1976). *Erik Erikson,* London: Collier MacMilla n.

Super, D., & Overstreet, P. (1960). *The vocational maturity of ninth grade boys*. New York: Teachers College.

Super, D. (1963). *Career development: Self-concept theory*. New York: College Entrance Examination Board.

Wessman, A., & Ricks, D. (1966). *Mood and personality*. Chicago: Holt, Rinehart & Winston.

9

EVALUATION OF THE CNS

Shirley W. Menard, M.S.N., R.N., and
Joan M. Wabschall, M.S., R.N.

Chapter Objectives

At the conclusion of the chapter, the reader will:

1. State the purposes of evaluation.
2. Discuss the different types of evaluation used to evaluate the role of the CNS.
3. Utilize an evaluation model or tool to evaluate the role of the CNS.

THEORETICAL PERSPECTIVES

Clinical nurse specialists have been in practice for more than 20 years. In that time, there has not been a tool developed to evaluate the CNS that encompasses all the many facets of the role. There have been numerous attempts to design such a tool, but to date, evaluation seems to be a problem area for most CNSs. This chapter will attempt to define some ways in which the CNS may be evaluated. It is not meant to be a definitive answer but rather a presentation of the current state of evaluation of the CNS as well as to give the reader some basis for her own evaluative tools.

For the purpose of this book, evaluation is a process of obtaining information concerning the role activities of the CNS for the purpose of self-growth and determination of cost-effectiveness. The development of a systematic evaluation plan requires an orderly approach (Figure 9.1). Clearly, one must have a purpose to be achieved by the evaluation process. For the CNS, the purpose may be a specific role function such as teacher. A statement of goals or outcomes is needed to determine if the purpose has been met. Next, the type of evaluation to be used must be decided. There are many types, such as peer review, self-review, and administrative review. All of these will be discussed in this chapter. The type of evaluation used will depend on what is being evaluated and what is the most recognized and efficient means of obtaining the needed information. Along with the type of evaluation chosen, one must also choose who will do the actual evaluation. Finally, there must be a specific time limit stated as to when evaluations are to take place.

Veney and Kaluzny (1984) define evaluation as "the collection and analysis of information by various methodological strategies to determine the relevance, progress, efficiency, effectiveness and impact of program activities" (Figure 9.2). CNS activities may be substituted in the above definition for "program activities". If one were to use this as a framework for evaluation: then one must look at each of the areas described by Veney and Kaluzny. Relevance would look at whether or not the CNS is needed. The progress section would track CNS activities. Efficiency would ask whether the CNS is the least expensive way to obtain results. Effectiveness looks at whether

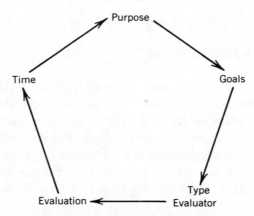

Figure 9.1. Model for evaluation.

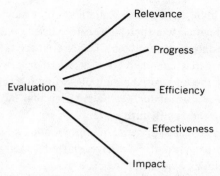

Figure 9.2.   Framework for evaluation.

objectives were or were not met. The CNS doing a self-evaluation might look at her goals to see if they were met. Finally, impact looks at the long-term implication of whatever is being evaluated. It is possible for the CNS to utilize the above framework for self, peer, and/or supervisor evaluation.

Nursing is under great pressure to be accountable to consumers for the care it provides. Professional standard review organizations (PSROs) have been around since 1972 and have been responsible for evaluating the quality of medical care. Nursing can also use the PSRO model and criteria established by ANA. In this way, nursing can be accountable and responsible for the provision of care. In the same way, the CNS can and should be responsible for her contribution to the quality of care given in her practice setting. If the CNS does not evaluate her practice, she may find that others will and that she has no practice at all because she has failed to show her worth.

The importance of the evaluative process cannot be underestimated, especially in light of the current state of health care economics. The CNS is constantly being asked to defend her impact on patient care. Prescott (1979) discusses one way to approach the cost-effectiveness issue: "Cost effectiveness is a relatively new approach to assessment of quality of care which focuses on expressing the end results or outcomes of care relative to the resources consumed to produce the outcomes" (p. 722). It is due to the rising cost of health care that providers are being asked to demonstrate their cost benefit and/or cost-effectiveness ratio to consumers. To institute a research proposal looking at whether or not the CNS is cost-effective, one must first look at financial and statistical findings. Financial costs are seen as total costs and then individual item costs. Statistical costs may involve looking at the portion of time devoted to a specific service such as patient care. The two costs (financial and statistical) are combined to find the total cost for a given item or service. Research can then look at whether providing the service involved costs less in the long run than not providing the service. It is through this type of a carefully formulated evaluative plan that the CNS may be able to prove her worth to the health care system.

Evaluation of nursing care per se is, of course, not a new subject. Methods for evaluation of direct patient care have existed for years. A part of the nursing process includes evaluation of care given. The difference between this evaluation and evaluation of the CNS seems to lie in the variety of roles a CNS assumes that have an impact indirectly rather than directly on the patient. For instance, the CNS, who in a consultative role recommends a specific plan of care cannot always be evaluated by the effect of that care on the patient. At times, the CNS must be evaluated for the indirect effect. Suppose that the consultee nurse carries out the plan appropriately — how does one evaluate the effect of the CNS? In other words, how much of the credit for the effectiveness of the plan on the patient goes to which nurses. It seems appropriate that we must develop a way to look at indirect care. If we can do this, we are in a much better position to document cost-effectiveness.

Evaluation of care appears to be a logical place to begin. Bloch (1979) talks about the three classic ways to evaluate patient care: structure, process, and outcome. Structure looks at the system. Process looks at the way in which care is given by a caretaker. Outcome looks at the results of that care.

Clearly, all three types of evaluation may be used at any given time. Structure evaluation of the facility will show how care is delivered. If there is only one CNS in a hospital, her effectiveness may be diluted by the structure and must be evaluated in light of the structure. The CNS must also be able to evaluate patient care using processes that may additionally be a way of evaluating the CNS. Naturally, patient outcomes such as decreased hospital stay are necessary to the CNS evaluation. Bloch (1979) goes on to describe a "process-related-to-outcome" evaluation that shows how the "actions of the providers relate to changes in the recipient of care" (p. 33). It is this type of evaluation that may assist the CNS to show that she truly makes a difference.

When one looks at process evaluation, one must look at the method of giving care. Hamric (1983) discusses the use of process evaluation to yield data concerning the ability of the CNS to perform her role functions. Hamric further discusses five types of process evaluations currently used in CNS evaluation: staff, administration, other health professionals, improvements in components of nursing process, and peer review (peer review will be discussed in detail later in this chapter). Evaluation by staff may be somewhat distressing to the CNS, but the personally and professionally secure CNS may find it very insightful and rewarding. Hamric and co-workers (1978) suggest an evaluation tool that uses a Likert-type scale to look at specific actions in light of their importance to the staff and the staff's view on how that action is performed by the CNS.

PRACTICAL IMPLICATIONS

Evaluation Tools

An adaptation of Hamric's tool may be used by the practicing CNS (Figure 9.3). The purpose of the tool is to define the importance of the various aspects of the CNS role to selected people with whom the CNS has contact. Additionally, it is hoped that this tool may be used as a self, peer, and/or supervisor evaluation of specific CNS performance.

When the tool is used as a self-evaluation, it may be necessary to have some type of documentation to help stimulate memory. One way of keeping track of weekly activities is by use of a form such as the one in Figure 9.4. This form is utilized by recording activities performed by the CNS under the appropriate role and day. The components of the four roles of the CNS—practitioner, teacher, consultant, and researcher—form the conceptual base of the tool. The roles were divided into components by using a series of statements or words derived from the CNS literature related to the role. A fifth area, professional attitude, was added to allow evaluation of the CNS as a professional.

The tool has two major categories, importance and evaluation. The "importance" section was designed to be given to all health care providers with whom the CNS has contact. The rationale for the importance scale is that it is difficult to evaluate or be evaluated until there is at least understanding, if not agreement, about priorities of the various roles and components. If what the CNS does is not seen as important by the people with whom she works, her role may not be valued. It is important to be sure that the importance section shows what the individual believes it is important for the CNS *to do*,

Thank you for agreeing to participate in this project on the role of the clinical nurse specialist (CNS). This questionnaire is important as a first step in evaluating the role of the CNS. Please fill in the following demographic data:

Position _____

Education _____

Age _____ Sex _____

Feel free to comment at the end of each section as I value your input. The sections are divided according to the various components of the CNS role. There are two sets of responses contained in the tool. The first set of responses concerns how important an aspect of the role is to you. The second set of responses is for you to evaluate my role as the CNS.

Please use the following key for completion of the responses for importance:
 N/A = Not applicable
 1 = Not important
 2 = Somewhat important
 3 = Very important

Please use the following key for completion of the responses for evaluation:
 N/A = Not applicable or not observed
 1 = Performs at an exceptional level
 2 = Performs at an acceptable level
 3 = Performs below acceptable level

I. Clinical practice	Importance	Evaluation
A. Provides direct care to selected patients.	N/A 1 2 3	N/A 1 2 3
B. Enhances continuity of care for patients in general	N/A 1 2 3	N/A 1 2 3
C. Is a patient advocate.	N/A 1 2 3	N/A 1 2 3
D. Expert at clinical decision making.		
E. Collaborates with other health professionals to assess, plan, implement, and evaluate patient care.	N/A 1 2 3	N/A 1 2 3
F. Provides effective health teaching to selected patients and families.	N/A 1 2 3	N/A 1 2 3

Comments:

II. Teacher	Importance	Evaluation
A. Teaches staff new procedures and skills.	N/A 1 2 3	N/A 1 2 3
B. Encourages discussion of patient care problems.	N/A 1 2 3	N/A 1 2 3
C. Identifies patient teaching needs.	N/A 1 2 3	N/A 1 2 3
D. Encourages staff to participate in educational offerings.	N/A 1 2 3	N/A 1 2 3
E. Contributes to learning of all health care students.	N/A 1 2 3	N/A 1 2 3
F. Develops and implements orientation programs.	N/A 1 2 3	N/A 1 2 3
G. Conducts nursing rounds and care conferences.	N/A 1 2 3	N/A 1 2 3

Figure 9.3. CNS role evaluation.

H. Identifies staff with potential for leadership or education and helps to develop this potential.   N/A 1 2 3   N/A 1 2 3

Comments:

III. Consultant

	Importance	Evaluation
A. Is approachable for help.	N/A 1 2 3	N/A 1 2 3
B. Listens to staff needs and concerns.	N/A 1 2 3	N/A 1 2 3
C. Assists staff to develop skills.	N/A 1 2 3	N/A 1 2 3
D. Assists staff to develop discharge plans for patients.	N/A 1 2 3	N/A 1 2 3
E. Works effectively with physicians and other health professionals.	N/A 1 2 3	N/A 1 2 3
F. Helps staff to find answers to clinical problems.	N/A 1 2 3	N/A 1 2 3
G. Assists administration on unit to identify staff needs and care problems and to find solutions for those needs and problems.	N/A 1 2 3	N/A 1 2 3

Comments:

IV. Research

	Importance	Evaluation
A. Carries out nursing research.	N/A 1 2 3	N/A 1 2 3
B. Assists staff to develop researchable questions.	N/A 1 2 3	N/A 1 2 3
C. Presents results of research to staff.	N/A 1 2 3	N/A 1 2 3
D. Encourages staff to read current articles and books related to specific areas of nursing.	N/A 1 2 3	N/A 1 2 3
E. Encourages staff to utilize results of appropriate, published nursing research.	N/A 1 2 3	N/A 1 2 3

Comments:

V. Professional Attitude

	Importance	Evaluation
A. Keeps staff informed of issues relevant to nursing and health care.	N/A 1 2 3	N/A 1 2 3
B. Role models what a professional nurse is.	N/A 1 2 3	N/A 1 2 3
C. Assists staff to evaluate the quality of care.	N/A 1 2 3	N/A 1 2 3
D. Keeps current in area of specialty.	N/A 1 2 3	N/A 1 2 3
E. Helps head nurse to develop standards of care and hold staff accountable for those standards.	N/A 1 2 3	N/A 1 2 3
F. Represents nursing in a favorable light to other disciplines.	N/A 1 2 3	N/A 1 2 3
G. Available to staff when needed.	N/A 1 2 3	N/A 1 2 3
H. Respects contributions of all health care workers to patient care.	N/A 1 2 3	N/A 1 2 3
I. Participates in community activities involving health care.	N/A 1 2 3	N/A 1 2 3

Comments:

Figure 9.3. *Continued.*

	Monday	Tuesday	Wednesday	Thursday	Friday	Saturday	Sunday
Practitioner							
Teacher							
Researcher							
Consultant							
Other							

Figure 9.4. Weekly report of activities.

not what the CNS *is doing*. The evaluation section may be used not only for constructive criticism but also to guide the CNS in goal formulation.

According to Colerick et al. (1980), the job description of the CNS can also be used as a method for evaluating the CNS. This "dual-purpose framework" may be delineated according to each hospital's needs as well as the needs of the individual CNS. A demonstration of this approach may be seen in Tables 9.1A and 9.2. The job description from Bexar County Hospital District is seen in 9.1, while a portion of an evaluation tool based on that description is seen in 9.2.

There are many process evaluation tools available in the nursing literature. One of these is Wandelt and Phaneuf's (1972) Slater Nursing Competencies Scale. This scale looks at all areas of nursing function and assigns a rating to each set. These rating scales evaluate the care *given* to the patient. They deal specifically with the nursing action involved rather than the effect of that action on the patient. The next type of evaluation is outcome evaluation. This type of evaluation looks specifically at the result of care as seen in behaviors or condition of the recipient of that care. Outcome criteria should be familiar to the practicing CNS as they are frequently a measure of student progress. Because outcome criteria are very measurable, a great deal of emphasis has been placed on specific outcome criteria. The difficulty with using only outcome criteria as an evaluative tool lies in the difficulty to show cause and effect. Many variables may have an impact on patient outcomes so it may be difficult to say that nursing action caused an outcome. The CNS who may be indirectly involved may have even greater difficulty showing her contribution to the outcome.

Process outcome evaluation is seen by Bloch (1979) as being the type of evaluation to which nursing must aspire. She lists five tasks that must be achieved in order to have a process outcome evaluation develop (pp. 33–34):

1. Development of a set of measurable outcome criteria specific to nursing.

2. Development of reliable and valid methods for measuring these outcomes.

3. Development of a set of measurable process criteria.

4. Development of reliable and valid methods for measuring the process of nursing care in all its various forms including both the physical aspects of the process as well as the psychosocial and cognitive aspects.

5. Testing of the various aspects of nursing practice in relation to patient outcomes, by applying process as well as outcome criteria.

TABLE 9.1.   Sample Job Description, Bexar County Hospital District[a]

Job Description: Clinical Nurse Specialist

SUMMARY

Function	As expert in specialized area of nursing, serves as guide to other personnel using skill in interpersonal relations to identify problems or barriers to individualized care and their solutions. Responsible for high-level patient care.
Scope	Areas of assigned responsibility may include broad areas of medical, surgical, psychiatric, obstetrical, pediatric, and rehabilitation nursing in BCHD and be directed to specific specialty areas of expertise; compliance with BCHD policies and procedures.

DUTIES

Typical	Gives direct care to selected patients and serves as role model of excellence in practice to others on unit. Evaluates nursing care requirements of patients, develops written nursing care plans, and evaluates care plan in operation and revises as indicated. Consults and makes rounds with medical staff, nursing personnel and other disciplines to achieve patient-directed goals. Teaches and demonstrates specific nursing care techniques. Plans and participates in team and multidisciplinary conferences. Participates in orientation, peer review, and staff development programs. Performs related duties as required.
Periodic	Identifies nursing problems in specific clinical area and conducts studies and research in systematic manner. Participates as active member of nursing and/or hospital committees. Prepares and submits regular and special reports as requested. Serves as nursing consultant to other medical areas in planning patient care.

SUPERVISION

Received	Responsible to Associate Administrator for patient care.
Given	None—advises, counsels, guides, and supports personnel in clinical management of care.

EDUCATION

Required	Master's degree in nursing. Licensed to practice in Texas. Maintains professional competency through participation in continuing education and other related training.

198

TABLE 9.1. *Continued*

Preferred	Master's degree with directly applicable specialized training.
EXPERIENCE	
Required	Master's degree in nursing. Licensed to practice in Texas. Maintains professional competency through participation in continuing education and other related training.
Preferred	Master's degree with directly applicable specialized training.
EQUIPMENT	
Required	Thorough knowledge of all instruments, equipment, and mechanical devices used in patient care in nursing specialty.
ACCURACY	Efficiency and accuracy in all phases of work.

[a] Any qualifications to be considered as equivalents, in lieu of stated minimums, require the prior approval of the Personnel Director.

TABLE 9.2. Sample Evaluation Tool, Bexar County Hospital District

Role	Criteria	Rating
Teacher	A. Shares case information with students and staff.	1 2 3 N/A
	B. Develops inservice programs particular to staff.	1 2 3 N/A
	C. Conducts and documents instruction to patients, staff and students.	1 2 3 N/A
	D. Demonstrates specific nursing care techniques.	1 2 3 N/A
	E. Participates in orientation of staff and students.	1 2 3 N/A

1. Exceptional
2. Average
3. Below Average

There is evidence that work has been progressing on these tasks, but the testing task still has far to go (Table 9.3).

Peer Review

The concept of peer review has been seen in medical and nursing literature since the 1960s. Peer review can be defined as the critical evaluation of one's work by a colleague equal in qualifications, expertise, and position. It is probably the type of evaluation, along with self-evaluation, that best meets the needs of the practicing CNS. Many times the CNS position is unlike any other position in the hospital, so it is difficult for someone other than a CNS to understand the position well enough to evaluate the person holding that position. Leibold (1983) states, "Peer review is particularly appropriate for the CNS, since this specialist has special responsibility for improving the

TABLE 9.3.   Process-Outcome Evaluation

Step	*Example*
1. Measurable outcome criteria	Postoperative patient does not develop wound infection.
2. Method	
3. Measurable process criteria	CNS teaches all personnel caring for patient, including nurses and physician, how to do postoperative wound care.
4. Method	
5. Testing	A research project with two groups of patients in which one group is taken care of by CNS-taught personnel and the other by a group of similarly qualified staff who have not had the CNS teaching knowledge of evaluation by research in the area of process outcome evaluation.

quality of nursing care and fostering the professionalism of nursing." Leibold further states, "CNS's who successfully learn to use peer review to improve their performance at the same time demonstrate the value of peer review to other nurses, who may in turn adopt the process to improve their own performance" (p. 221).

It is easy to see that peer review may be used for several different functions. Primarily, it is used as a tool for self-development, which is truly the goal of any evaluation. Because it is primarily a tool for development, the peer review should probably not be used as the basis for merit pay increases because of the difficulties inherent in evaluation of competitors for a monetary prize. Peer review may be used to strengthen the CNS group as a whole. When each member is able to increase her own development, it would follow that the group may also be strengthened. Peer review tends to promote trust between individuals because it is a tool used for self-growth and not generally for promotion or merit. There is less intimidation inherent in peer review when it is done in an appropriate manner. At times, evaluation can be a stressful event, but when done in a truly professional manner, it can be a growth-promoting event.

A model for developing a peer review system can be seen in Figure 9.5. The role functions are generally seen as those of practitioner, teacher, researcher, consultant, and change agent. Built into these functions is self-development for the individual CNS. The next step in the process is the development of criteria that test those role functions. Criteria development and development of a tool to test those criteria can be seen as part of the same step. Criteria are already available, such as those that appear in standards of care, job descriptions, and/or competencies. Also available are a number of

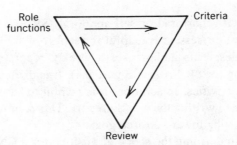

Figure 9.5. Model for peer review.

tools that measure the extent to which certain criteria have been met. The nursing care audit development by Wandelt and Phaneuf in 1972 reflects the quality of care given. It is not highly individual for CNS role functions and will need to be modified in order to utilize it for peer review of the CNS. Additionally, this audit presents a difficulty in that it is a closed-chart review and may not reflect the contributions of the CNS. It probably will be necessary to gather together many different evaluative tools and adapt them to the specific area of use. Table 9.4 presents a beginning outline of a tool that might be utilized. As shown, this tool is only a beginning. It illustrates some of the major points inherent in the practitioner role. The CNS who uses this type of evaluation would need to define the rest of her role functions in the same manner.

The peer reviewer selects the most appropriate number to describe how the person being evaluated is functioning. The area for comments allows the reviewer to offer suggestions for growth in those areas where growth is needed.

The final part of the triangle (Fig. 9.5) concerns the review mechanism itself. The performance of the CNS being reviewed must be evaluated in a nonthreatening atmosphere at regularly scheduled intervals. There should be a mechanism to document actions taken and also a method to evaluate the effectiveness of the review itself.

The use of peer evaluation then must be to limit evaluation to peer group, delineate objectives, facilitate individual accountability, review processes and outcomes, evaluate against standards, eliminate group self-protection, and show the cost-effectiveness of the group. When used in this manner, peer review is one of the most valuable of evaluative methods.

Self-Report and Self-Appraisal

The process of self-report and/or self-appraisal (SR/SA) is a good way to begin an evaluative process. It is helpful for self-growth to look critically at one's own activities. This author uses a weekly report sheet to organize thoughts in writing, or SR/SA (see Figure 9.4). It is difficult to remember 6 months worth of activities. In addition, it is helpful to have a copy of yearly goals available when writing the weekly report. This is of use in determining whether one is moving toward desired goals.

The first step in defining the scope of practice for a CNS is for the CNS to communicate a report of activities to nurse administrators in writing. In

TABLE 9.4. Outline for Peer Review

Use the following scale to complete this tool:
1 = Performed but not observed
2 = Performed below level of most CNSs
3 = Performed same as most CNSs
4 = Performed above level of most CNSs
5 = Not applicable to current role

Role	Criteria	Review	Comments
1. Practitioner	A. Use of process	1 2 3 4 5	
	Assessment	1 2 3 4 5	
	Goal setting	1 2 3 4 5	
	Interventions	1 2 3 4 5	
	Evaluation	1 2 3 4 5	
	B. Role model	1 2 3 4 5	
	Level of Skill	1 2 3 4 5	
	Knowledge of equipment	1 2 3 4 5	
	Interprofessional relations	1 2 3 4 5	
	Identifies issues	1 2 3 4 5	
	Resource person	1 2 3 4 5	
	Brings research to practice	1 2 3 4 5	
	C. Decision making	1 2 3 4 5	
	Patient care	1 2 3 4 5	
	Staff concerns	1 2 3 4 5	
	Management problems	1 2 3 4 5	

business, executives rely on annual reports to provide them with a profile of activities from various departments. The annual report is a tool to identify problems, trends, and progress. It is also used to analyze and evaluate the extent of programs and their effectiveness. By borrowing this concept of the annual report from business and incorporating it into the CNS role, the CNS is able to document the quality of care rendered and the achievements obtained through clinical practice. Due to the evaluative nature of the practice report, nursing administrators will find the practice report to be a valuable tool in determining compliance or noncompliance of the CNS with institutional role expectations.

The concept of a practice-based annual report for physicians has been described by McGuiness (1980). He believes that the annual report serves as an internal audit mechanism to ensure the maintenance of standards of care. By writing an annual report, one is monitoring the profession from within to assure that high-quality care continues over a lifelong professional career. Stevens (1980) acknowledges that the formation of a yearly report is an important activity for the nurse executive. Not only does it describe activities during a certain period but it also serves as a history of accomplishments. These views support the idea that a periodic activity report is a viable tool for the CNS to use in defining the role.

While very little information is found in the nursing literature to assist the CNS in preparing an activity report, guidelines for writing reports do exist. Papcum (1968) lists headings that can be used in a report by a nursing supervisor or nursing department. The CNS could incorporate the following headings suggested by Papcum (1968) into a CNS practice report: patient care activities, statistics, inservice education, problems, goals, and recommendations. Bernhardt (1978) suggests that the annual report contain a profile of the activities of the past year and give the results achieved, trends seen, and recommendations for improving service. Ewing (1979) believes that any standard report should contain an introduction that includes the purpose of the paper and a statement of the organization, a body, and conclusions. Conclusions should describe how the original objectives were met, include a summary and evaluation of the work done, and document the significance of the results.

In order to write a practice report, the CNS must incorporate these guidelines into a framework that can be adapted to the job description for her position as outlined by the institution in which she is employed.

A MODEL FOR THE CNS PRACTICE REPORT

The Wabschall model for development of the CNS practice report (see Figure 9.6) is based on the phases of the nursing process. However, before this framework can be used, the CNS must systematically document activities on a daily basis. Using the last 15 minutes of the day to jot down details is recommended. Activities can be recorded in a notebook using the categories outlined as major sections within the report itself or other tools, such as appointment books and time record calendars, may be used to record activities. Documentation of activities allows the CNS the opportunity to review the activities where a majority of time is spent as well as to maintain a goal orientation to practice.

Regardless of the tool used to document achievements, the task of writing the report will be less overwhelming if data are collected in an ongoing manner. If detailed records are kept, the activity report will almost write itself.

Job descriptions provide the role expectations for the CNS position. From a job description, the CNS can determine what initial goals need to be established. If job descriptions are not available, writing goals related to each subrole of the position is an appropriate place to start. Setting goals is an integral component of the practice report. Goals provide the structure for evaluation based on actual activities and outcome.

Within the Wabschall model, there are three columns labeled with terms that describe the phases of the nursing process. Each column contains boxes representing various parts in the process of report writing that correspond to the phases of the nursing process.

The column to the far left contains a box labeled Introduction. In developing an introduction to a report, the nurse is utilizing assessment and planning skills from the nursing process. Therefore, two separate boxes extend from the introduction. Within assessment, the CNS studies the existing job descriptions and guidelines in an attempt to understand the role expectations of the position. From this, role expectations are individualized into personal goals and strategies that the CNS believes will assist in achieving the desired outcome (see Figure 9.7). This preliminary process is crucial, as it gives the CNS a foundation to evaluate the original goals with actual activities and outcome.

Translation of role expectations and strategies into action is represented by the box labeled Summary of Activities. This section of the report corre-

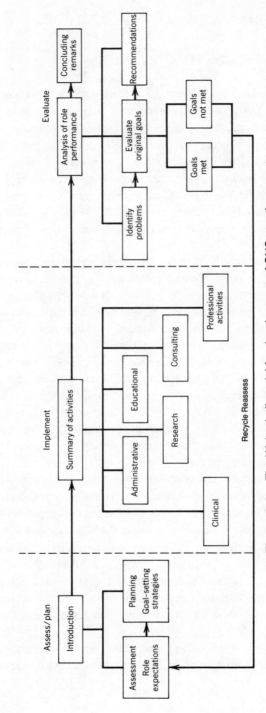

Figure 9.6. The Wabschall model for development of CNS practice report.

CLINICAL GOAL:

1. To promote excellence in clinical practice.

STRATEGIES:

1. a. To assist nursing staff in the development of holistic nursing care plans.
   b. To participate on the Nursing Standards Committee.
   c. To serve as a role model to nursing staff for planning and providing care to clients.
   d. To evaluate employees for the Clinical Promotions Program.

DESIRED OUTCOME:

1. a. By the end of the year, there will be an increase in the number of clients discharged with written care plans as part of the permanent record.
   b. As a result of my involvement with this committee, new and/or revised written standards of nursing care will be developed.
   c. By the end of the year, I will have provided care for a self-selected caseload of clients.
   d. Submission of employee performance evaluations will be made to the Clinical Promotions Review Committee.

FIGURE 9.7. Preliminary Planning—excerpts from a CNS practice report.

sponds with the implementation phase of the nursing process. It is within this phase of report writing that the CNS conveys the ways in which the role is enacted. Enumeration is used when writing this section of the report, which describes all activities. Enumeration clarifies a series of points and sets them in relation to one another. Enumeration also gives each point more visibility and therefore will have greater impact on the reader's mind (Ewing, 1979).

Six boxes are found under the summary of activities section that define the areas of practice and leadership addressed in this part of the report. Detailed activities to be documented include the areas of clinical involvement, administration, research, education, consultation, and professional activities. The column to the far right represents the evaluation phase of the nursing process. Within this phase one finds a box representing the section of the practice report entitled Analysis of Role Performance. Components of this section include three boxes: The first box represents problems identified within enactment of the role, the second box represents the evaluation of original goals, and the third box represents recommendations for future role enactment.

The process described in the first box (identification of problems) involves relating the obstacles and barriers that have impeded the enactment of the CNS role. These may be related to organizational constraints, interpersonal concerns, or conflicts within the CNS and the expectations associated with her role.

The second box involves evaluating the preliminary objectives and strategies formulated at the beginning of the process. To do this, the CNS compares the stated procedure to attain a certain goal with the actual activities. Desired outcomes and that which has transpired as a ᴇsult of the activities are compared. Goals are considered met or not met. Separate boxes extend from the evaluation box to represent this schematically. In both cases, reassessment occurs as new goals are formulated. Reassessment is shown on the model by the recycling/reassess arrow extending from goal evaluation back to the assessment phase.

Once the CNS has identified problems and evaluated original goals, recommendations are developed to deal with overcoming these problems and to reach new goals. Recommendations should stem directly from the first two components of the analysis of role performance section. Finally, concluding remarks are drawn that give the reader an overall picture of the success of the CNS. The conclusion is the final comment of the practice report; it corresponds with the evaluative phase of the nursing process.

Throughout the entire model, report writing is viewed as an ongoing process that requires the same assessing, planning, implementing, and evaluating as the nursing process methodology.

SR/SA can also be done on a verbal basis, but it is difficult to see trends if nothing is written down. If one gives a verbal SR/SA on a regular basis, such as in meeting with the Director of Nursing, one should always document what was reported. This can then be used to write a fuller report at 6–12 month intervals. The use of SR/SA and peer review are not only excellent evaluative methods but they are also a basis for self-growth in the professional role.

The case study following this chapter presents the use of SR/SA for evaluation. Each CNS must be willing and able to evaluate role and performance in order to be an accountable professional. It is possible that as we evaluate the CNS roles, we may also show the cost-effectiveness and productivity of the CNS.

BIBLIOGRAPHY

ANA peer review criteria mandated by HEW contact (NEWS). (1974, September). *Nursing Outlook*, **22**, 545.

American Nurses Association (1980, December). *Nursing—A social policy statement*. Code #NP-63, 35M. New York: American Nurses Association.

Bernhardt, J. H. (1978). Record keeping—Key to professional accountability. *Occupational Health Nursing*, **26**, 22–28.

Bloch, D. (1975, Winter). Evaluation of nursing care in terms of process and outcome: Issues in research and quality assurance. *Nursing Digest*, **3**, 32–41.

Boyan, D. (1981, Winter). Peer review: Change and growth. *Nursing Administration Quarterly*, **6**(2), 59–62.

Castronova, F. (1975). The effective use of the clinical specialist. *Supervisor Nurse*, **6**(5), 48–56.

Colerick, E., Bastnagel, P., Proulx, M., & Proulx, J. (1980, September). Evaluation of the clinical nurse specialist role: Development and implementation of a dual purpose framework. *Nursing Leadership*, **3**(3), 26–34.

Ewing, D. W. (1979). *Writing for results in business, government, the sciences, the professions* (pp. 114, 115, 242). New York: Wiley.

Girouard, S., & Spross, J. (1983). Evaluation of the CNS: Using an evaluation tool. In Hamric, A., and Spross, J. (Eds.), *The clinical nurse specialist in theory and practice* (pp. 207–218). Orlando, FL: Grune & Stratton.

Hamric, A. (1983). A model for developing evaluation strategies. In Hamric, A., and Spross, J. (Eds.), *The clinical nurse specialist in theory and practice* (pp. 187–206). Orlando, FL: Grune & Stratton.

Hamric, A., Gresham, M., & Eccard, M. (1978). Staff evaluation of clinical leaders. *Journal of Nursing Administration*, **8**, 18–26.

Leibold, S. (1983). Peer review. In Hamric, A., and Spross, J. (Eds.), *The clinical nurse specialist in theory and practice* (pp. 219–238). Orlando, FL: Grune & Stratton.

McGuiness, B. W. (1980). Why not a practice report? *Journal of the Royal College of General Practitioners*, **30**, 744.

Morath, J. (1981). Evaluation of the clinical nurse specialist. Paper presented at Second Annual National Clinical Nurse Specialist Conference, Cincinnati, OH, 1982.

Mullins, A. C., Colauecchio, R., & Tescher, B. (1979, December). Peer review: A model for professional accountability. *Journal of Nursing Administration*, **12**(9), 25–30.

Padilla, G., & Padilla, G. (1979, Winter). Nursing roles to improve patient care. *Nursing Digest*, **4**(6), 1–13.

Papcum, I. D. (1968). The annual report—An administrative tool. *Nursing Outlook*, **16**, 38.

Phaneuf, M. C. (1972). *The nursing audit: Profile for excellence*. New York: Appleton-Century-Crofts.

Prescott, P. (1979, November). Cost effectiveness: Tool or trap? *Nursing Outlook*, **27**,
722–728.

Reiter, F. (1966). The nurse-clinician. *American Journal of Nursing*, **66**, 274–280.

Stevens, B. (1976, February). Accountability of the clinical nurse specialist: The administrator's viewpoint. *Journal of Nursing Administration*, **6**, 80–82.

Stevens, B. J. (1980). *The nurse as executive* (p. 352). New York: Nursing Resources.

Taylor, J. W. (1974, June). Measuring the outcomes of nursing care. *Nursing Clinics
of North America*, **9**, 337–348.

Veney, J., & Kaluzny, A. (1984). *Evaluation and decision making for health services
programs*. Englewood Cliffs, Prentice-Hall.

Wandelt, M. S., & Phaneuf, M. C. (1972, August). Three instruments for measuring
the quality of nursing care. *Hospital Topics*, **50**, 20–28.

CASE STUDY: FORMALIZING SELF-EVALUATION THROUGH A CNS PRACTICE REPORT

Joan M. Wabschall, M.S., R.N.

I have found that the use of a CNS practice report that describes practice goals, strategies, and self-analysis of performance is an effective way to provide a complete and accurate account of a CNS's contributions and accomplishments. In addition, it provides a mechanism for evaluating the indirect effects of the CNS within the institution.

WRITING THE REPORT

The format I use for writing a CNS practice report is based on general principles of report writing. An outline for a CNS practice report is found in Figure 9.8.

I begin the practice report with a statement of how the report is organized and define the purpose of the report. Next, I summarize the content of the report in order to give the reader a quick self-appraisal of performance in each of the CNS subroles (clinical practice, administration, research, education, and consultation). In the section entitled Detailed Activities, I list the initial goals and strategies used to work toward the goals.

The detailed activities section is presented according to the subroles of the CNS role. For each subrole, a goal (or goals) is listed first, followed by enumeration of numerous strategies that were implemented. An example of a clinical goal is "to promote excellence in the care of pediatric surgical patients." Activities that

I. Introduction
II. Summary of activities
III. Detailed activities
Clinical area
Administrative area
Research and publications
Educational area
Consulting
Professional activities
Miscellaneous activities
IV. Analysis of role performance
Identified problems
Evaluation of original goals
Met
Unmet
Formulation of new goals
Recommendations
V. Concluding remarks

FIGURE 9.8.　An outline for the CNS practice report.

support that goal include written care plans, staff conferences surrounding patient care, or the direct provision of nursing care by the CNS as a role model. Examples of activities that would be included under the administrative heading would be coordination of patient care programs, participation in committee meetings, and assistance to head nurses in management functions. Research activities can include quality assurance projects or original research and may also include publications. Activities enumerated under the educational area should address three aspects: patient education (e.g., development of patient teaching tools), staff education (both formal inservices and informal demonstrations of nursing procedures or patient equipment), and continuing education undertaken by the CNS for personal and professional growth. Consulting responsibilities can be described in terms of contacts with other agencies or nurses in the community or in terms of interdepartmental consults within the hospital itself.

Since I began using the practice report 3 years ago, I have added a section under Detailed Activities that addresses contributions to the profession of nursing. This section was added because the CNS is viewed as a leader (or potential leader) in the nursing community, and such leadership expectations are often listed in job descriptions.

In addition, a last section dealing with miscellaneous activities was included to account for information on activities, such as hospital public relations efforts, that do not belong in any other section. The miscellaneous section can help diagnose the problems in time management. Since the CNS's time is more flexible than the staff nurse's time, the CNS is often pulled away from clinical practice to work on other projects. An overabundance of documentation under the miscellaneous category should alert the CNS to such a trend and prompt the CNS to refocus activities on components of practice that will have a greater impact on patient care. Since the role of the CNS is based on the subroles described in the detailed activities section, this section should be the lengthiest section of the report.

The fourth section of the practice report is an analysis that evaluates how well the CNS has done that which was set out to be accomplished. The original goals are evaluated for extent of achievement. If goals were met, new goals can be formulated with increasing levels of sophistication. Goals that have not been met or those that can remain pertinent are recycled, and new strategies are designed to achieve them. The new goals of the current practice report become the initial goals of the next report by which activities will be evaluated. Recommendations to address identified problems are listed prior to the concluding remarks. The report is submitted to the direct supervisor of the CNS prior to the annual employee appraisal date.

REFINING THE REPORT

The practice report described here as a self-evaluative tool has been utilized in clinical specialty practice with only minor revisions. I have found the report to be an effective method to convey contributions of a CNS to nursing administration.

A review of my past reports also indicates that my clinical practice has grown in regards to the level of sophistication of activities. This is a trend that can only be seen over time. A written practice report allows the CNS to evaluate subtle changes in a professional nursing career. This documentation of professional growth can be an added incentive to maintain the practice of writing the report.

The basic concept of a CNS practice report can be individualized and adapted to meet specific needs. Each CNS needs to evaluate the role as it is implemented in a particular institution and analyze personal enactment of clinical specialty practice. If more CNSs utilized such a report, we could begin to clearly define the scope of practice for CNSs.

CONCLUSION

The use of a CNS practice report is not the only way to evaluate specialty practice. Alternative options, such as peer review, have been discussed in the preceding chapter. Self-evaluation, however, is an important component of any evaluation.

CNSs contribute significantly to the standards of nursing care throughout the nation. Unless we are willing to devote some effort to document what it is we do, the value of the CNS to the institution and to the patient will continue to be questioned. The practice report is a component of evaluation that allows the CNS to describe the impact she has had on patient care and to gain recognition for the vital role she fulfills as a member of the health care team.

10

POSSIBILITIES AND PREDICTIONS

Shirley W. Menard, M.S.N., R.N.

Chapter Objectives

At the conclusion of this chapter, the reader will:

1. State the different models of joint appointments.
2. Define the difference between joint practice and independent practice.
3. Discuss the steps involved in establishing an expanded role practice.
4. Develop an understanding of the many opportunities open to the CNS.

Many exciting possibilities come to mind when looking at the future of the expanded role. From a variety of nursing areas, the CNS may choose the career that suits her best. This chapter will look at three of those challenging areas in depth: joint appointment, joint practice, and independent practice. The chapter will also briefly discuss other expanded role opportunities for the CNS.

JOINT APPOINTMENTS

The joint appointment in nursing has often been proposed as the ideal way to bridge the gap between nursing education and nursing service. The CNS is in a prime position to combine teaching and practice by negotiating a joint appointment between a university school of nursing and a service setting. The joint appointment, by definition, is a *shared* appointment between nursing service and nursing education. The division of time is negotiable, as is the division of payment. This section will discuss the history of joint appointments, types of joint appointments, positive and negative aspects of joint appointments, and how to negotiate such an appointment.

Florence Nightingale (1859) stated that the aim of her school was to *improve* the care of the sick. This gives a basis on which to build the CNS in a joint appointment. Christy (1980) discussed early schools of nursing in which there were few or no instructors. The students learned nursing from trained nurses within the hospital setting. The student nurse learned by watching the skill of others who practiced expert nursing care. It was natural that these skilled nurses should fill the gap in the education of students. During this period of time, there were no problems between education and service because the two were one. As the schools began to hire more instructors and the education of nurses moved into institutions of higher learning, a widening gap appeared between service and education. This gap has continued to widen until very recently, when there has been a move to put the most educated nurses back at the bedside. This is particularly evident in the advent of the CNS, who, with a master's degree in nursing, has shown that education truly enhances patient care.

As stated earlier, the joint appointment is shared between an institution of higher learning and a variety of service settings such as hospitals, community health agencies, and nursing homes. There have been efforts to establish the joint appointment on a wide scale in several institutions throughout the United States. In 1959, Dorothy Smith, at the University of Florida in Gainesville, began having faculty spend a portion of their time in direct patient care (Christy, 1980). In 1961, Case Western began a collaborative effort between the University and Hospital under a grant from the Kellogg Foundation (MacPhail, 1969). In 1972, two institutions began programs utilizing faculty in a unification model that is similar to but more than a joint appointment. One was at Rochester under Loretta Ford and the other at Rush under Luther Christman (Christy, 1980). It is helpful to compare these programs as they are somewhat different. At Case Western, the appointments may be given separately or they may be shared. Faculty may receive a clinical appointment from the hospital, while clinical staff may receive associate faculty status from the university. Additionally, there may be some faculty who are on a shared appointment status. Although this program does offer an extended faculty and more learning experiences for students, potential limitations are that it does not guarantee that faculty will practice and there is little flexibility of schedules.

At the University of Rochester, faculty are accountable for education and service. The clinician II is a master's-prepared faculty member who acts as a consultant to the bachelor's-prepared clinician I. The benefits of this model include an increased quality of patient care, faculty stay current in practice, and collegiality between nurses is promoted. The potential limitations of this model are the amount of faculty work load and the uncertain chance for tenure.

At Rush, under the leadership of Luther Christman as Dean and Director of Nursing, practice is a part of the job description for everyone. Two specific types of joint appointments are the unit manager and the practitioner-teacher. The unit manager is a master's-prepared nurse who directs clinical activities and participates in student education. The practitioner-teacher is a consultant for patient care, research, and teaching. The benefits of this model are an increased quality of teaching and care along with a reduced organizational hierarchy. Potential limitations include work overload, a need for very flexible people, and an inability to gain tenure.

The final type of joint appointment to be discussed is one currently in place between The University of Texas Health Science Center at San Antonio and Medical Center Hospital, one of the university's teaching hospitals. The appointment is 50% faculty and 50% CNS. The original appointment is with the School of Nursing, with a subcontract to the hospital. Currently, there are three such appointments with others being considered with different hospitals. As faculty, the joint appointee teaches one full course at the School of Nursing with clinical for that course occurring at Medical Center Hospital. In this way, the students see their teacher as a practitioner, and staff at the hospital see the clinical instructor as a practitioner who also teaches. In the other half of the appointment, the CNS is responsible for teaching, consulting, research, and practice in her area of expertise. Because of the support from the Dean of the School of Nursing and the Associate Administrator for Patient Care at the hospital, the joint appointees are able to choose the amount of time spent in various activities. In this way the CNSs are not as overloaded as other joint appointees have been, and burnout is less likely to occur. In fact, two of these joint appointees have been in the role for 5 years or more.

When one hears the words *joint appointment*, visions of heaven on earth tend to appear. The CNS who enjoys teaching and practice may jump for this type of appointment only to be disappointed to find that there are not enough hours in the day to adequately fulfill both jobs. A brief list of some positive and negative aspects follow:

Positive Aspects

1. The gap between service and education may be lessened.
2. The best educated nurses are at the patient's bedside.
3. Faculty practice is supported.
4. Staff is exposed to more research.
5. There is more promotion of collegiality between nurses.
6. Quality of care is enhanced.
7. Better learning is experienced by students.

Negative Aspects

1. The joint appointee may be overloaded.
2. Confusion between roles may be experienced.
3. There may be lack of rewards within academic setting.
4. Staff may compete with students for time.
5. In some instances, there is lack of authority in the service institution.

The positive aspects are self-explanatory and need no further discussion; however, the negative aspects need to be discussed in terms of either eliminating them or substantially reducing them. Overload may occur quickly if both institutions require 100% of the work week for their separate institutions. This requires the CNS to either not fulfill all that is expected or else to spend so many hours trying to do everything that fatigue and frustration quickly set in. The best way to eliminate this problem from occurring is to have the director of both institutions agree on paper as to the amount of activities required. This should be done with input from the CNS so that all can be clear on duties in each job. Additionally, the CNS must be able to say no to new activities if she is unable to add them to already standing duties. It is also useful for both agencies to realize that a joint appointment may be 50/50 some weeks and 60/40 at other times. The educational requirements are heavier at the beginning and end of semesters.

Confusion between roles may be the most difficult problem to solve next to overload. As faculty, one is treated in a certain way and is expected to do certain things. As CNS, one has other expectations and duties. It is sometimes hard to separate the two, and indeed at times, the roles do blend. One way to minimize this confusion is by having clearly defined duties in each role and by trying to have larger blocks of time for each role rather than short, interrupted time periods.

The lack of rewards such as tenure within the academic setting will not easily be overcome. Some faculty have strong feelings toward those faculty who are not always available in the educational setting. When a CNS has a joint appointment, there is not as much time to spend in scholarly discussions with one's academic colleagues. Because of this, the CNS in a joint appointment may be seen as an outsider in academia. This type of treatment is changing as more faculty have become involved with practice and as more joint appointments are created. There are more deans and directors who are supporting the concept of the joint appointment, which also helps to legitimize the role and make the rewards better. It is still not possible to obtain tenure while on a joint appointment, but at least recognition as a faculty person is accorded.

A final problem area occurs within the service area when the CNS is in a staff position rather than a line position. It is generally necessary to negotiate the joint appointment between the two institutions. The first step is to discuss the possibility of such a venture with the dean of the educational facility and the director of nurses of the service institution. The best argument one can use for the joint appointment is the bridging of the gap between education and service. Once an agreement between the two institutions is made, the CNS must decide which institution will hold her contract. It appears best to have one institution be the hiring agency, with the second institution having a subcontract. In this way, benefits and salary may be better. The choice as to which institution should hold the primary contract should be carefully studied by the prospective CNS. Many times the decision is made by comparing salary, benefits, and degree of autonomy.

The CNS should be a partner in the refinement of the job description for both institutions. Negotiations about time commitments should also be made at this time. This is especially important so that both institutions are aware of the total time commitments of the joint appointee. The service institution must understand that during school semesters, the CNS may spend more than 50% of her time in teaching. The educational institution must understand that during school breaks, especially summer, more time will be spent at the service institution. Because duties will differ depending on the institutions, specific duties for each part of the appointment will not be discussed. For a sample of an initial job description, see Table 10.1.

In negotiating a contract, where there are not already specified rewards, the CNS must remember to ask for vacation and sick benefits, conference travel, professional journals, and other benefits. A decision must be made about how these benefit costs will be shared. This must be decided early, not after the contracts are signed. A major problem in joint appointments appears to be a lack of preliminary planning. Problems frequently encountered must be solved prior to accepting the job, and a method for solving problems that occur later must be specified. If care is taken during the negotiations for a joint appointment, there is a good chance that it will be successful.

JOINT PRACTICE

Joint practice is practice with another health care professional. Although there are many professionals the CNS may work with, the most common arrangement is with a physician. The initial decision to work *with*, not *for*, a physician must be approached much as one approaches the joint appointment. It is important that one carefully investigate the practice prior to signing a contract. The CNS must be sure of her status within the practice and her contribution to decision making.

In order to begin negotiations for a joint practice, the CNS must be able to market her skills. She must be prepared to tell the physician just exactly what she can add to the practice. Additionally, she should have some idea what this will do for the practice in a monetary sense. The CNS should also be well prepared to discuss facts showing the CNS as an effective and revenue-producing partner. Recent journal articles supporting this position may be beneficial.

In negotiating salary and benefits, the CNS should calculate the minimum salary she will accept as well as a reasonable optimal figure. Increments should also be discussed with intervals for raises specified. Benefits should include vacation and sick leave, conference travel, professional dues and journals, a mileage allowance if the CNS will be doing much home visiting, malpractice insurance, and any other items that can be negotiated.

Evaluative periods should also be specified at the outset, with 6 months and 1 year the most common times. This is needed so that both CNS and physician can evaluate the impact of the CNS on the practice and also gives a time when honest input can help improve the practice. It usually takes about 6 months for the CNS to settle in and begin to have an impact on the practice. If she is evaluated sooner, there may be a false impression that she really is not adding much to the practice. If too long a period of time goes by, the CNS and physician may allow problems to be compounded before approaching them. In addition to formal evaluation sessions, there needs to be a weekly time set aside to problem solve those areas that have arisen during the week.

One difficulty that can occur when a CNS is in a joint practice concerns hospital visiting privileges. If the CNS is to really be a partner in the health care team, she must be allowed to participate in hospital care. The kind of hospital privileges will vary from state to state and from hospital to hospital. In some areas, the CNS may visit patients in the hospital, write orders, and do histories and physicals. In other areas, the CNS may not even be allowed official visiting privileges. Some agencies have a credentials committee that reviews curriculum vitae/license/references from nurses. Once the nurse is "credentialed," she may visit/care for/write in charts and write orders that the physician countersigns. This needs to be discussed and handled early in the negotiations. The concept may be new to the hospital and may need to be thoroughly presented to the hospital board. It may be necessary to look at state law and/or the hospital policy in order to show the legality of the CNS. It may also be necessary to engage a lawyer to protect the CNS's interests. It is vital that the CNS approach and resolve this difficulty early.

Joint practice is certainly an exciting possibility for the CNS who wishes to practice in a truly collaborative manner with another health care professional. The CNS must choose her practice partner carefully and negotiate a contract that will give her rewards—professional, monetary, and personal.

INDEPENDENT PRACTICE

Perhaps the ultimate in practice is the establishment of an independent nursing practice. The CNS who chooses this direction must plan carefully prior to the start of such a practice so that she is not bogged down by unforeseen problems. Independent nursing practice is not a new concept. It has been around since the days of early private-duty nursing. The establishment of an independent nursing practice is once again becoming a focus of debate be-

Table 10.1. The University of Texas School of Nursing at San Antonio, Joint Agency–Faculty Appointment

A joint agency–faculty nursing position would enable qualified clinical nurse specialists to engage in teaching, research, and patient care while simultaneously bridging the gap between the concerns of nursing service and the goals of nursing education.

All candidates for joint appointees should have a master's degree in nursing with a minimum of 3 years clinical experience in the area of specialization. The candidate must meet requirements for a school of nursing faculty position as well as requirements for the agency's clinical specialist position. Appointments may be 50–50 or any other combination of effort mutually agreed upon by nursing education and nursing service.

In the school of nursing the candidate would hold a faculty appointment and receive faculty rank. The individual would be responsible to the dean of the school of nursing. In the service agency the candidate would receive an appropriate title (clinical nurse specialist or clinical pediatric nurse specialist) and would be directly responsible to the Assistant Administrator for Nursing (or equivalent position).

The candidate will have the freedom to arrange his/her time schedule so the needs of students, staff, and patients can be met. This may mean blocks of time devoted to either service or education activities or the utilization of weekends, evenings, or nights to be with staff, patients, or students. The scope of activities should be delineated by the candidate and approved by both nursing service and education.

The following areas of activities would encompass the overall job description of the candidate. Specificity and a time frame for accomplishment would be the responsibility of the candidate.

Faculty	*Service*
1. Serve as role model to students by providing exemplary nursing care to patients.	Serve as role model to nursing and medical staff by providing exemplary nursing care to patients.
2. Interpret and support School of Nursing philosophy and programs.	Interpret and support nursing service philosophy and goals.
3. Orient students and faculty to area of specialty.	Orient new nursing staff to care of patients in specialty area.
4. May participate in selected classes in areas of specialty for	Participate in the improvement of patient care through staff education

Table 10.1. *Continued*

graduate or undergraduate students.	and active participation in giving patient care (selected by CNS).
5. Supervise undergraduate and/or graduate students in the clinical area of specialty. Assist students in assessing, planning, and intervening in patient care activities. Evaluate student performance. Serve as consultant for faculty in area of specialty.	Participate in direct care and serve as consultant for staff nurses in the area of specialty.
6. Participate selectively on faculty committees. Meet with coordinator and faculty group when appropriate.	Participate on selected committees and programs in relation to specialty area and interdisciplinary efforts.
7. Identify researchable clinical nursing problems and initiate or participate in development of research ideas.	Identify researchable clinical nursing problems and initiate or participate in development of research ideas.

cause consumer groups and government are looking for alternative methods of health care delivery while organized medicine argues that such practices violate the Medical Practice Act.

Neal (1982) discusses the different factors that make up the pattern all people follow in starting their own business. Displacement or a feeling that it is time to do something different may follow some type of situational crisis. Many people who start their own businesses experience control of life as being within themselves. They dislike being controlled by others. Credibility or the belief that you can start your own business is another factor that is necessary to succeed. Finally, resources, financial and otherwise, will be needed to open an independent practice.

When starting to consider an independent practice, there are ways to obtain the needed advice and support. Neal (1983) states that there are five ways to bridge the gap from employee to self-employed. One can join a *networking group*. This will give the CNS the opportunity to meet and talk with other entrepreneurs. Still another way is to observe a *role model* who has her own business. Find a *mentor*; another nurse who can be supportive to the CNS and give guidance. Joining a *professional business organization* may give the beginning independent the group support she needs. Last but not least, the nurse entrepreneur needs to attend *seminars or workshops* on starting a business. Keeping abreast of books on finances, office management, and so on may also be of assistance.

The initial step (see Figure 10.1) in beginning an independent practice is to find out exactly what the state Practice Act says nursing is authorized to do. It is also necessary to check the Medical Practice Act to determine what constitutes the practice of medicine. The Board of Nurse Examiners will know what type of certification (if any) is required to open such a practice. In some instances, no further education or training beyond a basic nursing education may be necessary. In some states, a master's degree in nursing is necessary for an expanded role practice. It is vitally important to know the law concerning medicine and nursing in your state.

A second important step is to define the services the CNS will provide to her clients. These should be stated in writing and be clearly visible to potential and/or actual clients. If the CNS is planning to see clients who may need what may be construed as medical care, she must have a list of physicians to whom she can refer clients needing care she cannot provide. A list of protocols to follow may also be needed, and these should be approved by a physician. Some states require that the protocols also be approved by the Board of Nurse Examiners in the state. It may be necessary to draw up a contract between a physician and the CNS so that the CNS will have adequate medical

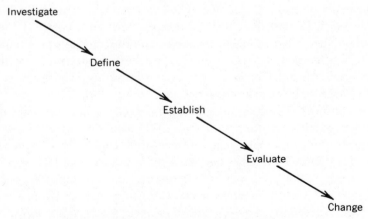

FIGURE 10.1 Steps to independent practice.

backup should it be needed. It is vitally important that the CNS remain within her practice act.

The next step involves the actual establishment of the practice. The CNS may work out of her home or rent office space in a building. Expenses that may be incurred prior to actually opening the practice include rent, equipment, supplies, phone, advertisement, and paid help. Rental on office space can be very high in desirable locations. The CNS may wish to look at other areas to begin her practice. A small vacant shop may prove to be a bargain. Only very essential equipment should be bought or leased, that is, items for physical assessment, chairs, desk, and medical supplies. Paper and other secretarial supplies must be obtained, and a phone line must be installed. Marketing the practice is essential if the business is to succeed. This can be done by means of flyers, advertisements in local newspapers, radio spots, and word of mouth. One may also send out professional letters with business cards enclosed. Referrals can come from physicians, other nurses, satisfied clients, and friends. Be very clear in the advertising that a professional nursing practice is being opened. Confusing statements may lead to litigation. Paid help is really not a necessity at first, but the CNS will eventually need someone to type, file, and answer the phone. One place to obtain someone to help may be through the local high school if there is a work-study program.

In establishing the practice, the CNS should choose a name for the practice that helps to define it. The CNS must decide if the practice is to be incorporated or not; to do this may require the help of an attorney. Additionally, the business may need to be registered, and licenses may need to be obtained. A tax number must be gotten from the Internal Revenue Service, and an accounting method must be established. A budget that is reasonable and able to be followed must be determined quickly. The budget should be realistic and include all of the possible expenses (rent, utilities, salaries, equipment, insurance, marketing). (The Small Business Association provides various kinds of assistance in setting up a small business.) Overestimate rather than underestimate cost. A recommended accountant may provide invaluable and needed expertise. It is essential that a commitment be made to the practice, and a limit should be set beyond which the CNS cannot continue if the practice is not successful. This period should not be less than 1 year.

Establishing a practice also means establishing rates of payment from clients. It is generally wise to charge a reasonable amount rather than undercharging because then there is a tendency to rush people through so more can be seen in a day. In addition, people tend to equate price with quality so that undercharging may have a negative effect on business. The fee schedule will depend entirely on services provided, but a basis for that schedule can be found in the rates of other health care providers in the area. If the state allows nurses third-party reimbursement, the insurance code may set the fee schedule. A practice will take time to grow and become successful. It also takes money to establish a practice and keep the CNS in creature comforts, like food and clothing, during the establishment phase, which may take up to 2 years.

It may be necessary to take a loan to fund you through the initial period. Banks, savings and loans, or small business agencies are possible places to secure such a loan. The CNS may also find it better to work part time in an institution while she is setting up an independent practice. Money is definitely an issue to consider when starting an independent practice.

An evaluation of the practice should be done every 6 months for the first 2 years. Items to be considered include cash flow, patient satisfaction, numbers of referrals, and CNS satisfaction. At each 6-month evaluation, plans should be made to change those areas of the practice that seem to be a problem. The CNS should realize that it takes time and patience to establish an independent practice; it will not occur overnight.

Finally, it is the responsibility of the CNS in private practice to publish and share her successes and insights with other nurses. All too often, nurses who are successful neglect to share with others. Journals such as *Nursing Economics* are an excellent medium in which to communicate the entrepreneurship of nurses.

The three types of CNS practice discussed are by no means the only avenues open to an ambitious and creative CNS. An astute CNS may be in demand as a representative for drug and equipment companies. The advent of DRGs has forced health care to devise alternatives to physician-only care. A groups of CNSs could get together and form a PPO (preferred-provider organization) to offer low-cost preventive health care to various companies while referring illnesses to physicians. Still another opportunity for the CNS is as a case manager either hired by a company or contracted to a company to audit health care costs and recommend more efficient ways of providing care. The future is bright for an enterprising CNS who has expertise to offer and the wherewithal to pursue her dreams. The future for the CNS looks very promising. The three case studies that follow describe how one CNS established a joint appointment, how another CNS set up a practice with two other health professionals, and how a CNS has a new career as director of a group of CNSs.

BIBLIOGRAPHY

Allen, P., & Turner, D. (1982). Perinatal dimensions: A successful beginning. In Neal, M. (Ed.), *Nurses in business* (pp. 71–88). Pacific Palisades, CA: Nurseco, Inc.

Appelbaum, A. (1978, July). Commission leads way to joint practice for nurses and physicians. *Hospitals*, **52**, 78–81.

Baker, N. (1983, December). Entrepreneurial practice for nurses: A response to Hershey. *Law, Medicine and Health Care*, 257–259.

Campbell, E. (1970, March). The clinical nurse specialist: Joint appointee. *American Journal of Nursing*, **70**(3), 543–546.

Campbell, M. T., & Owen, E. C. (1982). A joint psychiatric practice. In Lynch, M. L. (Ed.), *On your own: Professional growth through independent practice*. Monterey, CA: Wadsworth Health Sciences Division.

Chamorro, T. (1981, July 15). The role of a nurse-clinician in joint practice with gynecological oncologists. *Cancer*, Supplement, 622–631.

Christman, L. (1979, March). Statement of belief regarding faculty practice. *Nursing Outlook*, **27**(3), 158.

Christy, T. (1980, August). Clinical practice as a function of nursing education: An historical analysis. *Nursing Outlook*, **28**(8), 493–497.

Devereux, P. M. (1981, May). Essential elements of nurse-physician collaboration. *Journal of Nursing Administration*, **11**, 19–23.

Diers, D., & Molde, S. (1983, May). The new gatekeepers? *American Journal of Nursing*, **83**(5), 742–745.

Elliot, D. (1983). Unified role of educator, clinician, research—Why not all three. In Beal, J. (Ed.), *Advanced practice in pediatric nursing* (pp. 255–263). Reston, VA: Reston.

Fasano, N. (1981). Joint appointments: Challenge for nursing. *Nursing Forum*, **20**(1), 72–85.

Frederickson, K. (1982). A multidisciplinary group practice. In Lynch, M. L. (Ed.), *On your own: Professional Growth through independent nursing practice* (pp. 139–165). Monterey, CA: Wadsworth Health Sciences Division.

Hayden, M. & Rowell, P. (1982). Hospital privileges: Rationale and process. *Nurse Practitioner*, **1**(7), 42–44.

Hershey, N. (1983, December). Entrepreneurial practice for nurses: An assessment of the issues. *Law, Medicine and Health Care*, 253–256.

Kuhn, J. (1982, October). An experience with a joint appointment. *American Journal of Nursing*, **82**(10), 1570–1571.

MacPhail, J. (1980). Promoting collaboration/unification models for nursing education and service. *Cognitive dissonance: Interpreting and implementing faculty practice roles in nursing education.* (pp. 33–36). New York: National League for Nursing.

Mills, B. & Free, T. (1984, May/June). Nursing faculty practice. *Pediatric Nursing*, **10**(3), 212–214.

Neal, M. (1982). The socialization of nurses. In Neal, M. (Ed.) *Nurses in business* (pp. 3–16). Pacific Palsades, CA: Nurseco, Inc.

Nightingale, F. (1859). Notes on nursing: What it is and what it is not. London: Harrison and Sons.

Rose, M. (1984, May). Laying siege to hospital privileges. *American Journal of Nursing*, **84**(5), 612–615.

Steele, J. E. (1981, May). Putting joint practice into practice. *American Journal of Nursing*, **81**(5), 964–967.

Willian, M. K., Weinberg E., Burnett, R., & Olmsted, R. (1978, March). The pediatric nurse associate: A model collaboration between medicine and nursing. *New England Journal of Medicine*, **13**(298), 740–741.

CASE STUDY: A JOINT APPOINTMENT
Eleanor Adaskin, M.A., R.N.

The purpose of this case study is to describe the early development phases of the CNS role in an urban, public, 850-bed acute care teaching hospital in midwestern Canada. Central issues in the change process and some of the role's achievements and problems will be reviewed.

PLANNING FOR THE CHANGE

The introduction of the CNS role occurred rapidly, as a part of several objectives of the Director of Nursing. Because she wished to place resources for clinical excellence near the bedside of patients, she had recently decentralized both administrative and continuing education personnel. The CNS role was seen as a way to concentrate clinical expertise so that nurses and patients could draw on-the-spot help with care and learning. To supplement the clinical knowledge available to all nurses, the director hoped over the next 5 years to create CNS positions within every specialty department of the hospital.

Since I was at that time the first master's-prepared supervisor and very much interested in investing more time clinically, the director decided to open the first position in psychiatry, my area of specialization. Concurrently, I was asked to embark on a trial year of joint appointment with the local University of Manitoba School of Nursing, assuming clinical supervision for a group of baccalaureate nursing students in psychiatric-mental health nursing. One-third of my time was to be for the university, and two-thirds for the hospital CNS role. The goals for this venture were for nursing education, service, and research to become more closely linked through a role that crossed the traditional divisions between them. It was exciting to embark upon these multiple, interlocking change processes. Not surprisingly, however, we encountered both benefits and problems in trying to accomplish our complex goals.

BUDGET CONSIDERATIONS

Canada's totally tax-funded health care system might seem the ideal place to begin a role founded on the ideals of quality of care. Unfortunately, however, the CNS position was created at a time of cutbacks in local government funds for health care. Consequently, with no new monies to be gained, funding for the role was "pieced" together from existing amounts accrued as a result of previously unfilled nursing positions in the Department of Psychiatry. With little time to acquaint the nursing staff with the possibilities of the CNS role, the change was initiated. Staff nurses' attitude, though open in principle, was dampened somewhat by the heavier work loads they experienced due to the cutbacks in staffing throughout the hospital. The CNS role may have seemed somewhat a "frill," given the pressures with which they coped daily. However, perhaps because they and I have enjoyed a generally positive relationship over my 2 years in the supervisor role, the nurses were more receptive and accepting of the change than they might have been had an outsider been as rapidly injected into the system.

REPORTING LINES

After much discussion, it was decided that the goal of on-the-spot coordination of efforts toward clinical excellence would be best served by keeping the reporting lines for the CNS role localized within the Department of Psychiatry. Consequently, a triad was visualized with the new supervisor (formerly head nurse of the inpatient unit), the new head nurse, and the CNS forming a closely integrated group. They would work together to assess clinical and teaching needs for nurses within the department and to plan, implement, and evaluate the ways in which the triad could unify efforts to meet these needs. The CNS would report to the supervisor but, for practical daily purposes, remain closely connected with the head nurse and staff. Annual objectives for the CNS, mutually agreed upon by the CNS and the supervisor, would form the basis for an annual performance appraisal.

Communication lines of a more informal, "staff" type were visualized from the CNS to the Director of Nursing. It was expected that the CNS would be able to assist with hospitalwide issues, projects, and consultations and for these purposes be in direct communication with the director. Further "staff" relationships would exist between the CNS and the director and staff of the Continuing Education Department within the hospital as a whole for coordination of efforts in educational matters. The Director of Continuing Education would monitor the quality of educational projects designed by the CNS.

SALARY ISSUES

The CNS had been paid previously at the supervisor level. However, there existed an administrative hospital policy that no worker could earn as great a salary as the person to whom she reported. In order to bring her salary in line with that policy, the CNS's preexisting salary was held constant while hospitalwide nurses' salaries underwent increases. Eventually, the CNS salary was released approximately halfway between the head nurse and supervisor levels. The differences in educational level for the three positions were recognized (only the CNS position required or had a master's degree), but pay scales within the hospital system were built on principles of administrative hierarchy, where the worth of management-level positions was related to the number of workers over which a leader held direct or indirect "line" responsibility. The CNS had no one reporting directly to her, so the breadth and depth of her responsibilities was not clearly measurable by these criteria.

The department-level salary, though founded on the ideal of on-the-spot availability in each clinical department, did not reflect the breadth of functions the CNS was requested to perform across the hospital system and in the community. In this respect, the choice of a "staff" rather than a "line" relationship and department versus hospitalwide reporting lines for the CNS position resulted in some practical limitations in salary. Such salary policy could be viewed as needing new guidelines that would find ways to assign appropriate monetary value to both staff and line leadership. However, in the initial period, when the CNS position was vulnerable to overall financial shortages, there was tacit agreement to work on building and providing the worth of the role before trying to achieve all the structural answers.

MULTIDISCIPLINARY RELATIONSHIPS

Within our hospital, a period of increased multidisciplinary staffing and collaboration was already underway when the CNS role was introduced. These groups had welcomed my clinical and teaching interests when I had been a supervisor in the Department of Psychiatry. The role of CNS was of even greater appeal to them, since they visualized further opportunities to share clinical problem solving on a daily basis, engage in innovative program planning, and pool efforts for teaching material common to all of our disciplines. Such material included group and family dynamics, interviewing skills, psychosocial assessments, and so on. Additionally, they were appreciative of the availability of another experienced therapist with whom to conduct therapy or exchange peer feedback, which furthered our mutual clinical skills. Our shared knowledge base and conceptual and clinical backgrounds made immediate teamwork easy.

Whereas in many settings nurse therapists are viewed with suspicion by psychiatrists and other disciplines, I was fortunate to meet positive and relatively egalitarian attitudes. Since family therapy was my major clinical focus, I was pleased to receive referrals from the psychiatrists during my efforts to have family assessments become as routine for patients as individual admission interviews. With a gradual increase in psychologists and social workers able to conduct family interviews, family work was shared among us all. With the support of the Medical Director of Psychiatry, we formed a multidisciplinary Family Clinic that grew from 3 to 10 members over a 5-year period. This group provided service, education, consultation, and research functions. All of us held other positions within the department but gave a few hours a week to working with or teaching about families.

The springboard for this project was the demonstration and teaching of family therapy to the fourth-year medical students and later the psychiatric residents. We were gratified at the opportunity to model interdisciplinary teaching for students who, for the most part, were otherwise taught only by members of the medical faculty. In recognition of this role, our Chief of Psychiatry arranged formal appointments for Family Clinic members to the Faculty of Medicine at the university. This added to the growing legitimation and support for the CNS role at the multidisciplinary level.

HOSPITALWIDE CONSULTATION

Requests soon arrived from nurses in other departments who wished consultation on psychosocial problems related to both patient and staff issues. A kind of "troubleshooter" role developed for the CNS. Patient consultations included seeing a confused and oddly behaving elderly patient on a medical unit; a pregnant young Nigerian woman who would not comply with her nursing care; an unwed teenager who had just lost her baby; a surgical patient who seemed to be prolonging her recovery; and many others.

Among the staff were communication difficulties: between nurses and physicians in high stress areas; among nurses within a unit and their head nurse; and by whole groups of nurse managers in coping with decentralization or interdepartmental conflicts. The 40-member head nurse group, the 15-member supervisor group, and the 18-member continuing education group each requested consultations or workshop sessions. Generally, these dealt with issues in communication, self-esteem, and the change process. Delivering health care in a complex high-tech hospital was proving a demanding task, in which the services of the psychosocial CNS were sought for high-touch (people-oriented) interventions.

Additionally, the CNS was called upon by the Director of Nursing to participate in various committees and task forces in the hospital. Ladder systems of advancement were being suggested for teacher-practitioners as well as for administrative nursing staff. The possibility of tying pay scales to levels of practice, though attractive from a clinical excellence point of view, held potential conflicts within the union structure in the hospital. The CNS was asked to help gather input from all levels of nurses by serving on the Staff Management Committee, a vehicle for resolving actual and potential problems between staff nurses and nursing administration. Again, the knowledge base of the psychosocial CNS (including the change process, professional nursing issues, group dynamics, and basic human relations) seemed to find application at many levels as the nursing division worked to promote change at a hospitalwide level.

CONSULTATION AT COMMUNITY LEVEL

From the community came other types of consultation and teaching requests. The Continuing Education Department of the local university asked the CNS to teach family assessment to community health nurses whose original education had not provided sufficient family theory and practice. A multidisciplinary 12-week evening course was given and then repeated several times due to the enthusiastic response. Many drove 2 or more hours after a work day in outlying communities in order to improve utilization of their regular visits to families through increased knowledge of family systems. In addition to nurses, a few psychiatric occupational therapists and a family practice physician attended. Course members noted this course as a rare opportunity to improve mutual understanding between groups within and outside of nursing.

Other community responsibilities included service on various mental health and nursing research boards and committees. Interdisciplinary and intranursing collaboration from these contacts often laid the base for networks that could be called upon by the CNS to assist hospital nurses who needed community resources. Liaison with the local university was reinforced through both the joint appointment role and by board and committee service. In some ways, it became difficult to distinguish where professional community service in general began and where the community role of the CNS ended.

This spread of service beyond the walls of the hospital was sometimes a point for discussion when the management/CNS triad was trying to determine how the

CNS should apportion her working time. Often, daytime work crept into evening hours, while community service called upon some of the CNS's workday hours. The concept of a nine-to-five job was rarely applicable for this fluid and complex role.

BREADTH VERSUS DEPTH ISSUES

Given the widening circles of requests for consultation and service, the psycho-social clinical specialist was faced with the dilemma of how to establish priorities for division of her time. The original intent of on-the-spot consultation to staff nurses and their patients was ever more difficult to attain. Although the path to nursing excellence in general was being pursued by interventions at the broad system level, these commitments often made it difficult to sustain clinical focus at the unit level. It became clear that early visions of applying the role mainly to nurses and patients in the Department of Psychiatry were not to be realized if multiple broad functions were simultaneously performed. Sorting through these dilemmas was part of the evolutionary process of developing the role.

Although the original role description for the CNS contained reference to most of the functions eventually sampled, it did not help us to decide what proportions of activities to choose at any particular time. Often reassessment arose as one or another group of expectations collided. The early "Cinderella" phase of rosy hopes that the CNS would fit a multitude of glass slippers soon faded. We realized that eventually several people would be required. Among those discussed were: a roving troubleshooter for the hospital nursing department at large; a hospitalwide psychosocial liaison nurse for other clinical departments (or CNSs for individual areas); a staff counselor; and on individual units, teacher-practitioners who could assist the CNS to plan and implement staff learning programs and patient care improvements.

The direct clinical role of the CNS, though imagined as a central part of my work, in truth shrank to perhaps 2–3 hours a week. Since other responsibilities so often involved my absence from the clinical area, sustained primary nursing contacts with inpatients were impossible. It became more feasible to serve outpatients and families coming in for weekly scheduled therapy. However, even these interviews sometimes collided with unexpected calls for a sudden administrative meeting or patient consultation elsewhere in the hospital. Such collisions highlighted the various value systems lying behind the ideals of the role.

When and how much should one commit to direct patient care, or teaching, or the overall "excellence goals" being pursued by the entire nursing group within the hospital? No easy answers were available, and whichever choice of activity we made, certain other activities had to be relinquished or delayed.

One is often warned by time management specialists that it is important to be able to say no. The difficulty with following this advice is in achieving agreement on which request should be refused. Since most requests for the CNS's service were important and valid, it was often difficult to choose which to decline. The triad attempted to negotiate answers to such intradepartmental dilemmas at our monthly meetings.

Proportioning of hospitalwide and communitywide involvement required consideration of long-term rather than short-term benefits to the hospital. In many cases, advantages of improved working relationships within the hospital and community were "felt" rather than measured. However, the question of how to keep a depth of clinical focus while achieving these broad benefits was never satisfactorily resolved. One solution was simply to keep rotating the multiple role functions, giving higher priority to some areas within a particular 3- or 6-month period.

Since, in general, a centrifugal force seemed to spin the CNS away from unit-level function, we eventually became aware that other teacher-practitioner personnel would be needed who could participate with the CNS in planning educational and clinical improvements but who could be more continuously present on the units for implementation of such programs.

This solution was implemented just as the CNS was funded to leave for doctoral study. Some of her psychiatric department functions were divided between two new baccalaureate nurses with teaching experience. One took over the future development of a competency-based orientation and staff development program. She was given the mission of creating self-learning packages that staff nurses could use to advance their nursing excellence in a levels of practice project in psychiatry. The other took over the direct teaching of specific psychiatric nursing programs such as handling aggressive behavior. The broad functions of hospital and community service were not specifically reassigned for the period of the CNS's absence, although some of these were absorbed by other nursing personnel. It was proposed that the two new members and the CNS work together upon her return from educational leave. With this combination, it was hoped that both breadth and depth of involvement could be achieved.

SUMMARY AND RECOMMENDATIONS

As a result of our experience in implementing the CNS role for the first time in our hospital, we learned a number of things. First, this type of important change would benefit from a longer period of planning, wherein all levels of nursing and other disciplines could work together to create realistic understanding of the possibilities and limitations of the role. The phenomenon of Cinderella and the multiple glass slippers needs to be addressed long before the CNS makes her appearance and is found to possess only the customary number and size of human feet. When one person proves insufficient to meet all the imagined functions, everyone may be left somewhat disillusioned. For hospitals planning such a change, it would be helpful to bring in an established CNS consultant who can assist the hospital to prevent some of the pitfalls encountered repeatedly in such roles.

A systems approach to consultation would involve all levels of nursing, along with the disciplines who will be most involved in the future CNS's functioning, including some representation from the community. The use of CNS case study discussions at this time can give opportunity to consider the role strains and role collisions common to such positions. Value systems that lie between each group's expectations become clearer when actual situations can be problem-solved through discussion. In the group's attempt to reach agreement on the CNS case situations, those who most value the direct clinical role can dialogue with those who visualize the CNS as filling mainly educational functions. Those who consider multidisciplinary planning or overall quality monitoring can exchange viewpoints with those who value hospitalwide or community-level liaison functions for the CNS.

Out of such discussions, more realistic expectations can emerge as to the impossibility of any one CNS in filling all potential needs. As a result, the group can arrive at a concensus as to which of the glass slippers they most want the new Cinderella to fit. This helps both the drafting of the role description and the selection of a CNS who will be suited for the chief functions of the role.

There do not appear to be any easy answers to the issues of salary and reporting lines. If line rather than staff power is chosen for the CNS, the incumbent will need to balance additional administrative responsibilities along with the other functions discussed. Line power allows for clearer salary scale placement within the traditional heirarchy but may not allow for the nonthreatening types of nutrient and integrative power that is basic to functions such as consultation, counseling, and objective troubleshooting. Power for another and with another are sometimes difficult to mix with direct power over another person. Additionally, it may be difficult to find an incumbent who has both the ability and the wish to combine executive, clinical, educational, and consultation functions.

Reporting lines can be complex for CNSs choosing staff types of positions. This person, though designated as holding responsibility for her functions, must accomplish most goals through influence rather than through direct authority over others. Obviously, interpersonal and interprofessional relationship skills will be of the utmost importance, as is the person's credibility as a competent practitioner, teacher, and consultant.

Who will evaluate the CNS in these multiple autonomous functions? Who will know the depth or breadth of her ability as practiced in each role segment? Evaluation of a specialist can be problematic since the definition of the role usually acknowledges the ability to practice at the growing edge of advances in an area of specialty. In our situation, evaluation was accomplished through the supervisor's and CNS's review of annual objectives that had been mutually agreed upon. This process, however, could never draw in all the widening rings of function throughout the hospital and community. It must be recognized that all evaluations are partial, not sampling the total of a person's performance but only selected aspects such as written yearly objectives. It would have been desirable if the informal reporting line between the CNS and the hospital's overall Director of Nursing could be included during the evaluation process, considering the number and scope of projects undertaken by the CNS in developing the role. Although these wider projects generally arose separately from the CNS's psychiatric department objectives, regular evaluation and feedback as to the director's opinion of the effectiveness of the CNS's participation in such projects would be valuable and appropriate.

Issues of breadth versus depth will perhaps always be a source of role strain and time management problems for the CNS. The role entices all who devise or occupy it. It is tempting to the clinically oriented person who hopes the role can provide opportunity to practice one's expertise in clinical depth. It beckons the planners with visions of all-encompassing benefits in quality enhancement and broad institutional problem solving. However, it seems unlikely that both breadth and depth can be sustained steadily by any one role occupant. The challenge lies in choosing a human-size glass slipper and the right Cinderella to fit it.

CASE STUDY: INDEPENDENT PRACTICE
Barbara Carlile-Holmes, M.S.N., R.N.

A viable alternative for the delivery of ambulatory care services is available to the CNS via a private practice. I have defined the term *private practice* as the delivery of nursing care to clients on a fee-for-service basis. How does a nurse begin a private practice? The following is an explanation of the planning and implementation of a private practice in nursing in a southwest metropolitan city.

During my final semester in graduate school, I was enrolled in a class entitled Psychiatric/Mental Health Nursing in a Community Setting. The graduate students in this class were allowed to choose the site for their clinical setting as long as the setting fell within the criteria of the university's standards. The setting was to be one that delivered services to clients but that preferably did not have a nurse in its employ. We were to assess the need for the role of a nurse in such a setting and propose the implementation of a professional nursing role. I chose as my setting a holistic health center directed toward patients with cancer, owned and managed by a clinical psychologist. In addition to the psychologist, the center employed two psychotherapists, one part-time dietitian, one part-time fitness expert, and two part-time secretaries. It rapidly became evident that the skills of a nurse would greatly enhance the services offered to clients. I recommended to the psychologist that he allow a nurse to establish a private practice in conjunction with his practice. We discussed this concept, and it was decided that I would establish a private nursing practice within his center.

My first step was to obtain legal advice. I consulted with a former attorney at the Texas Nurses' Association who was able to clarify further the Texas Nurse Practice Act. Through this consultation, I obtained clear-cut guidelines as to those activities that fell under screening and those that fell under diagnosis in this state. Any time a nurse practices nursing she must be acutely cognizant of the rules and regulations governing the practice in that particular state. This is true regardless of the practice setting: hospital, home health care agency, or private practice. Through my legal consultation I found out that nurses can now not only perform a physical examination but may also order lab work pertinent to the individual patient. The lab work is classified as a *screening* tool, that is, the nurse can utilize the lab work, such as the CBC or chemistry profile, to establish normal from abnormal. A diagnosis based on this lab work, however, still falls under the realm of medical practice. My attorney then recommended that I speak with the president of the local medical society to inform him of my plans for establishing a private nursing practice. This was done in a collegial manner, not in a permission-seeking one. I presented to him my plans for establishing a private nursing practice. His first response was that I was "not practicing nursing." This gave me opportunity to explain to him the full realm of nursing practice in today's world. The conversation ended on a positive note, with his having a better understanding and a new respect for the expanded role of the nurse.

I also consulted with two nurse colleagues in Dallas, Texas, who had established their own private practice. Their practice was not directed toward patients with cancer. However, I was able to obtain much information from them regarding the business management of such a practice. They were able to give me much direction regarding size of an office, need for a secretary/receptionist, and necessary equipment.

I then established a contract with the psychologist. The contract provided for my use of one office and for partial secretarial help. I agreed to pay the psychologist 10% of my collected (not billed) monies for this space and service. As my practice grew, his percentage would increase to 30%. The psychologist and I jointly employed a graphic artist to devise a logo and name. Building signs, brochures, stationery, and business cards for each of us were all designed incorporating the logo and name of the practice. Additionally, newsletters carrying articles on good health practices were designed and mailed to selected groups of people.

I received referrals from a variety of sources: patients, nurses, and physicians. The majority of referrals for patients with cancer came from private medical oncologists in the community. However, I also saw patients who were self-referred and interested in improving their overall health. These patients did not have a diagnosis of cancer but were given information regarding exercise, nutrition, and stress and a cancer-preventive life-style. I was quite amazed at the number of self-referrals I received from patients. This communicated to me the need for more nurses to be in private practice.

There were other health care professionals who were available for referral through this center. These included registered dietitians, physical therapists, and physicians. Contracts with each of these disciplines were established between the psychologist and each of them. I was then able to refer patients to each of these specialists.

The majority of services that I provided to patients and families with cancer were for education and support. Patients were generally referred to me for education regarding their diagnosis, treatment options, and coping with cancer on a daily basis. Individual psychotherapy was also available for these patients.

I initially devoted 4–6 hours per week to this private practice. I arranged to see patients during the day, in the evenings, or on weekends. During this time, I was also working full time in a local university, and had to limit myself to a maximum of 6 hours per week.

I established a payment procedure that was based on a fee for service of $50.00 per hour. A sliding scale was also devised, however, based on the patient's individual financial status. At the time of this writing, third-party reimbursement for nurses is still not available in Texas.

Several types of tax considerations were involved in setting up this private practice. Taxable income varies according to the amount of deductable expenses. An accountant familiar with small-business laws should complete the annual tax form. The city and county taxes that were assessed on my practice and the building consisted of an arbitrary assignment of dollar values on commercial buildings. This resulted in the main problem area I encountered. I owned one desk and one chair within my office. The assessment made on my personal property was $10,000. It took 6 months and numerous letters and phone calls to correct the inappropriate assessment. The tax assessment procedure is based on the assumption that the proprietor will take the responsibility of reputing any unfair tax assessment. The most limiting problem area that I have encountered in my private practice is that of inadequate reimbursement. If third-party reimbursement for nurses existed nationwide, many components of the health care system could benefit. Koltz (1979) describes the benefits of a private nursing practice noting that the client would benefit by receiving immediate and direct health care. Physicians would benefit by referring appropriate clients to the nursing private practice, thereby confining more of their time to diagnosis and treatment of disease. Hospitals could discharge patients earlier. Insurance companies could pay the private practice nurse at lower, yet just, rates. The government would also benefit as a public insurer. Another problem area is that of balancing time commitments. It has been difficult for me to maintain this practice while working full time, but the rewards have been worth the effort. A very different type of problem encountered was the promotion of unconventional types of treatment by other "holistic health centers."

I have found that the challenge and fulfillment associated with this endeavor is unmatched by any other aspect of my career. Private practice offers a challenging career opportunity to the nurse with entrepreneurial interests.

REFERENCE

Koltz, C.J. (1979). Why private practice? In Koltz, C.J. (Ed.), *Private practice in nursing*. Germantown, MD: Aspen.

CASE STUDY: DIRECTOR OF CNSs, A NEW ROLE
Annie Johny, M.S., R.N.

At St. Paul's Medical Center in Dallas, Texas, utilization of the CNS was begun in the early 1970s. During that period, there were only two CNSs, and they had been hired into staff positions. They reported to the Director of Nursing for a short time and then to the Nursing Director in charge of Quality Assurance and Patient Classification Systems. In the 1980s the need for more CNSs was identified due to increasing numbers of patients with multifaceted and complex health problems. In order to meet the needs of these challenging patients, a systems approach was utilized to develop a dynamic, integrated, comprehensive, and multidisciplinary program. The nuclei of this program were the seven CNSs in Arthritis, Cardiovascular, Diabetes, Maternal–Child, Oncology, Psych–Mental Health, and Pulmonary.

During this time of change, the functions of the Director of Quality Assurance were incorporated into other job descriptions, and the position was deleted. The CNSs were then asked to report to the Assistant Administrator for Nursing. I was practicing then as the diabetes CNS. Functioning in a staff position afforded the freedom to make nursing decisions for quality care because there were few administrative tasks to bog me down. Authority and power came from my knowledge and clinical expertise in diabetes. Resistance to the role of CNS came from many factions in the beginning, but improved patient outcomes helped to overcome that resistance.

One major difficulty was identified when the CNS reported to the Assistant Administrator for Nursing. Due to a variety of responsibilities, the administrator was not able to meet with CNSs on a regular and frequent basis. It seemed appropriate to create a new position so that the group of CNSs could receive the support and direction they needed to fully implement their own roles. Initially, a part-time director of CNSs was appointed from the ranks of the CNS group. This arrangement did not work because of the same time constraints as other administrative persons. In 1984, a full-time Director of CNSs was appointed.

My position as Director of CNSs gave the CNS group the advantages of both staff and line positions. The director functioned in a line position and was able to voice CNS concerns at the administration level. Each CNS functioned in a staff position in her respective area. The Director of CNSs was responsible to the Assistant Administrator for Nursing.

The Director of CNSs negotiated and contracted with administrators and department directors for activities done by the CNS group in their area. Activities included being directly or indirectly involved with planning, implementing, and coordinating programs offered in the various departments. The cost for the CNSs was charged to the cost centers that utilized their expertise. This brought revenue to the CNS group.

St. Paul's Medical Center also operated a number of ambulatory care centers in the Dallas–Ft. Worth metroplex. The CNS group provided health education and screening to the patients in these centers. The Director of CNSs contracted with these facilities for the CNS time and also for the cost of producing educational materials.

The Director of CNSs functioned as a troubleshooter for the group, which allowed the individual CNS to be more productive. Programs and projects were accomplished with more expediency because there was someone who could help the CNS problem solve difficult areas. CNSs could get questions answered and issues clarified more quickly because the director was available. This reduced the frustration level for the CNS, which led to increased productivity and creativity.

In summary, the role of CNS director created a more positive working experience for the CNS group. Additionally, they enjoyed higher visibility because the director could market the CNS role. The director position required someone who understands the role and function of the CNS, is assertive, is skillful at negotiating, and diplomatic. It is a large task for one person but also offers great rewards.

INDEX